Helene Byrne

Exercise After Pregnancy

How to Look and Feel Your Best

with a Foreword by Kim Mulvihill, M.D.

Celestial Arts

BERKELEY / TORONTO

CELESTIAL ARTS

Post Office Box 7123, Berkeley, CA 94707   www.tenspeed.com

Celestial Arts titles are distributed in Canada by Ten Speed Canada,
in the United Kingdom and Europe by Airlift Books, in South Africa by Real Books,
in Australia by Simon and Schuster Australia, in New Zealand by Southern Publishers Group,
and in Southeast Asia by Berkeley Books.

Cover and Text Design by George Mattingly, GMD/Berkeley.
Photographs by Don Tuttle.   Illustrations by Helene Byrne.

LIBRARY OF CONGRESS CATALOGING-IN-PUBLICATION DATA

Byrne, Helene, 1956–
Exercise after pregnancy : how to look and feel your best / Helene Byrne.
p. cm.
ISBN 1-58761-004-3
1. Postnatal care. 2. Weight loss. 3. Exercise for women. 4. Physical fitness for women.   I. Title.
RG801 .B974 2001
618.6—dc21

2001002625

First Printing 2001
Printed in the United States of America
1 2 3 4 5   05 04 03 02 01

ACKNOWLEDGMENTS

The creation of a book is a collaborative process, and I am indebted to all the talented individuals who helped me realize this dream.

Thanks to Cariad Hayes, who helped shape and structure my initial ideas into a coherent and marketable format. I wouldn't have had the guts to take on a project of this scope without your guidance and expertise.

Thanks to Tom Southern and all the folks at Celestial Arts for seeing the potential of my work and taking the risk of publishing a first-time author.

Thanks to Sarah Nawrocki and Judy Bloch for their insightful and careful editing.

Thanks to George Mattingly for his elegant book design.

Thanks to Don Tuttle and his assistant Joe James for their precise and artistic photography.

Thanks to my beautiful postpartum models, Romy Falck, Barbara Parker, Ilana Seidel Horn, Soo Ko, Eileen McCullough, and Carol Keufer, for taking the time out of their busy new-mother lives to learn, rehearse, and photograph the exercises.

And mostly, thanks to my dearest husband John, and my most wonderful son Jason, for filling my life with love.

L

It is understood that any exercise system should be followed with care and sensitivity.

Please consult with your doctor before beginning this program or resuming any other exercises after pregnancy and childbirth.

CONTENTS

FOREWORD

by Kim Mulvihill, M.D.

Not long ago pregnant women were discouraged from exercising. Doctors feared physical activity might harm mother and child—diverting precious blood flow away from the uterus and baby. But our views on exercise and pregnancy have evolved. A recent study, for example, found that women who exercised regularly during pregnancy had slightly bigger babies, slightly bigger placentas, and no harm to either. Today exercise is considered part of a healthy lifestyle and part of a healthy pregnancy.

Pregnancy changes your body profoundly. To meet the needs of your developing baby you produce more blood and your heart works harder to pump it. Pregnant women require up to twenty percent more oxygen, and as the uterus grows larger and larger, breathing gets harder and harder. Hormonal changes lead to loose ligaments, especially in the hips and pelvis (to make childbirth easier). Even the curvature of your spine changes, shifting forward and throwing off your center of gravity. And yes, pregnancy also means weight gain. These are normal physiological changes, but they make it harder to exercise and impossible to reach your fitness peak.

After delivery your body begins a slow process of recovery. If you exercised regularly during pregnancy, you're a step ahead. But no matter how fit you were before or during pregnancy, you need to go slowly now. Many of the physical changes of pregnancy (including loose hips) last four to six weeks after delivery, so it's best to resume activities gradually. If you had a difficult birth, a Cesarean section, or if there were complications after delivery, wait a little longer before starting to exercise. Be sensible and listen to your body to know how much is too much. Always check with your doctor before starting any exercise program.

Helene Byrne offers a unique approach to reconditioning after pregnancy. Simply put, her program works from the inside out. The focus is on balance, core strength, and realigning the spine—elements basic to getting fit after having a baby. The program helps restore muscle tone and strength, while emphasizing good posture. It teaches good habits to last a lifetime. Reconditioning is not about dropping 35 pounds. In fact, it's not at all about dieting. It's about getting fit for the rest of your life. And it makes tremendous sense.

So how do you fit exercise into an already hectic schedule? When a good day with a new baby means getting a shower before dinner, it isn't always easy to exercise your sleep-deprived body during your few free minutes of the day. But it's worth the effort. Exercise lifts your spirits, helps you relax, and improves your strength and stamina. You'll feel better and sleep better. And you'll find it easier to do all the activities of a new mom.

Exercise has to be a priority and part of your daily routine. Yes it takes commitment. It also takes planning, compromise, and loads of flexibility. Keep in mind that staying fit over the long haul is more important than getting into shape right after birth. So, choose the fitness level appropriate for you as you follow the excellent program Helene Byrne has devised for *Exercise After Pregnancy*. Physical fitness is essential to good health. You owe it to yourself and you owe it to your family.

INTRODUCTION

Several weeks after my son was born, I felt ready to start exercising again. As a dance and fitness professional, I was keenly interested in getting back into great shape as fast as humanly possible. I started with Kegels (contractions of the pelvic floor muscles), crunches to work my abdominals, and other traditional toning exercises. But after several frustrating weeks, my body didn't feel or look any better. I was experiencing a lot of muscular tightness, and I was developing what my husband and I jokingly referred to as my "Jason muscle" (named in honor of my son)—painful spasming of the muscles around my shoulder blades. My lower back felt compressed, and no amount of stretching gave effective relief.

My body had become a stranger to me. Everything felt disorganized and disconnected. Nothing worked well. I realized that profound systemwide changes had occurred in my skeletal alignment and that my body was functioning completely differently than it had before pregnancy. To find out what was going on I gave myself a series of muscle functioning tests, the same ones I use to develop a personal training program for a new client.

Much to my dismay, my previously fine-tuned body was functioning as if I'd had no training at all! It was as if my years of dance and fitness had evaporated. I had lost all functional control and stability. It was a humbling experience.

The results of the functioning tests revealed that I needed to reestablish the fundamentals of good neuromuscular technique. Not only did I need to rebuild my pelvic floor muscles and abdominal wall, I also needed to retrain my abdominals to function as stabilizers so that I could maintain good form during exercise and daily activities (in fitness jargon we call this "dynamic stability" or "functional core strength"). Fortunately I had the professional skills to tackle the job.

I developed a system of exercise focused on alignment and functional core strength. Just weeks after I began this less traditional approach I began to see dramatic results. My abdominals began to flatten and move back toward my spine. My lower back no longer ached and once again became long and elastic. The spasms in my upper back muscles abated, and my shoulders no longer hunched forward.

I began to feel like myself again. I stood taller and had more energy. Lifting and carrying my baby and all the requisite gear became easier. My sleeping patterns improved, and I could handle the stresses of motherhood and baby care in a more relaxed manner. I could more fully enjoy being with my precious newborn.

Three months after giving birth I ran into a neighbor who exclaimed, "Wow! You've lost all your pregnancy weight already. You're so lucky!" Of course I hadn't really—I still had twelve pounds and three dress sizes to go. But what she saw in me was good carriage of the spine. I looked good, and felt good, because I had reestablished good alignment.

In fact, many people said that they thought my body looked more attractive than before pregnancy. This was a surprise because, like all new mothers, I was plumper, softer, and (for the first time) voluptuous. I realized there was beauty in this kind of body too. By accepting that my body was just how Mother Nature intended it to be, I could let go of what I thought my body should look like and appreciate what I had: a fit and beautiful "mommy body." Looking at my old clothes hanging in the closet was no longer devastating.

New motherhood is one of life's most exhilarating, joyous, and rewarding experiences. It's also one of the most challenging, tiring, and frustrating—it doesn't have to be a backbreaker too. This book offers a fast, safe, and effective program to restore the body to optimal functioning after pregnancy. It will have you looking and feeling your best.

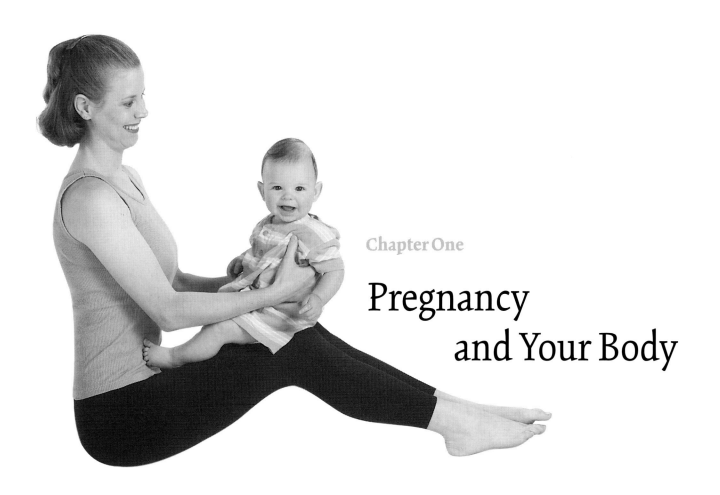

Chapter One

Pregnancy and Your Body

NEW MOTHERHOOD is thrilling, challenging, mind-numbingly exhausting, frustrating, and overwhelmingly wonderful—sometimes all in a single hour.

The postpartum months can feel like a roller-coaster ride at the best and the worst of times. During pregnancy the body has nine long months to adapt to the changes it's going through. After childbirth women's bodies change much more dramatically. The uterus shrinks rapidly and the milk factory begins operation. Nothing seems to work the way it did. Shoulders and lower backs ache. Episiotomy or cesarean stitches hurt. Sleep deprivation fuzzes the brain. And because newborns demand so much time and attention, it's all too easy to overlook the need for physical rehabilitation.

More than ever, women today understand the pivotal role of fitness in health and wellness. And we want to pass on to our children the physical and psychological benefits of a healthy lifestyle. Pregnancy and childbirth were once considered to be the beginning of the end for a woman's body. It was thought that women could never be as strong or fit after pregnancy. They were encouraged to accept their weakened state as an inevitable consequence of childbirth.

But this theory doesn't hold up. Muscles respond to exercise in the same way after childbirth as before. Reconditioning after pregnancy is not only possible, it's essential for optimizing maternal health. It helps us meet both the physical and psychological demands of parenthood.

Pregnancy and childbirth place extreme stress on the body. Whether you had a home or hospital birth, vaginal or cesarean, medicated or natural, your body has been through one of life's most strenuous events. Your internal organs, muscular system, connective tissue, bones, and joints have been taxed to their limits. Many changes occur in the spine, connective tissue, and muscular systems. Deviations in align-ment coupled with extreme laxity in the ligaments and the abdominal wall create an imbalanced system that lacks dynamic stability (the ability to maintain good form during movement) and functional control. The physical demands of motherhood—lifting and carrying the baby, and dealing with heavy diaper bags, strollers, and car seats—further stress an already weakened system, leaving you vulnerable to pain and injury. No wonder so many new moms suffer from lower back pain, muscle spasms, and related problems.

To be at your best, you must restore your body to an adequate level of functioning. Postpregnancy reconditioning not only prevents complications such as urinary stress incontinence and back pain, it also provides an important psychological boost. When your body is functioning well, you look and feel good. The demands of motherhood are easier to handle. And if you must return to work shortly after childbirth, the need for reconditioning is even more urgent.

The body recovers from many aspects of pregnancy naturally. The uterus, stimulated by breast-feeding, contracts to close to its former size in about six weeks. The body's ligaments slowly return to their former length and elasticity over three to six months. But muscle tissue does not rebound so easily. Without direct stimulation, muscle tissue will not return to its former length, strength, or functional capability. And without exercise, muscles atrophy and weaken. The cliché "Use it or lose it" is accurate.

During the second half of pregnancy the body's center of gravity shifts. As a counterbalance, the pelvis tips forward and the pubic bone moves backward, increasing the curve of the lower spine. In response, the upper back increases its curve, giving the chest a caved-in look. The neck curvature also increases, making the head slide down and forward.

When the pelvis and spine are misaligned, some muscle

groups are stressed and tighten, and as a result must work harder to maintain the upright position. Other muscle groups are underutilized and weaken. By the third trimester, most women find good posture nearly impossible to maintain, especially by day's end.

The body also produces elastin and relaxin, hormones that, as their names imply, relax and lengthen the ligaments in preparation for childbirth. Ligaments, which connect bone to bone, are the body's passive restraint system and provide stability to the joints.

The abdominal muscles stretch to an astonishing degree and become unavailable for spine support. After birth, the abs look, feel, and function more like pudding (no one ever warns you about this) and can no longer effectively support the spine and the internal organs.

During a vaginal birth the pelvic floor muscles (which run from the tailbone to the pubic bone) stretch to their limits. It's amazing how much the birth canal and pelvic floor open during childbirth to accommodate the baby's head. These muscles must be reconditioned to prevent serious complications such as urinary stress incontinence, loss of sphincter control, and uterine and/or bladder prolapse, a serious condition where one or both organs collapse onto the vagina.

The cesarean birth has its own problems. Because the uterus and abdominal wall have been surgically cut, reconditioning must wait until the sutures have healed, a process that takes four to six weeks. However, once the stitches have healed, you do not have to worry about injuring the incision sites during exercise. Scar tissue is very strong. You can begin postpartum exercises as if you had a vaginal birth. And because the baby has not passed through the birth canal, the pelvic floor is usually intact. Some of the problems associated with the pelvic floor (tearing, episiotomy pain, anal sphincter stretching or tearing) are much less severe or avoided entirely.

After pregnancy the body must be retaught to maintain good alignment during movement and muscle groups must be retrained to function synergistically. Muscle groups are like pulley systems: groups that have become overly tight, or hypertonic, pull the bones out of ideal alignment. Overly lax, or hypotonic, groups cannot counterbalance these forces, so the body continues to distort into the undesired posture. This, in turn, increases the amount of compression on the vertebrae and intervertebral discs, and because of the increased laxity of the ligaments (which normally help support the vertebrae and maintain the curve of the spine) the spine is particularly vulnerable to injury. And what we experience, of course, is pain.

The reestablishment of good alignment, functional stability, and balance of opposing muscle groups is the most important concept in postpregnancy exercise. Isolating muscle groups with the goal of increasing muscle density (as most traditional toning regimes do) simply isn't good enough, especially after childbirth. These exercises do little to develop synergistic functioning. You can think of muscles as being instruments in an orchestra. Each must learn its own part, but in order to create music they must all learn how to play together, as one voice. So, too, with the body. Strong limbs with a weak or nonintegrated center are a recipe for injury. In both everyday life and competitive sports the spine must be able to absorb the force of impact without twisting out of alignment. A healthy, strong, supple spine can be developed only when alignment, stability, core strength, and elasticity are the cornerstones of an exercise program.

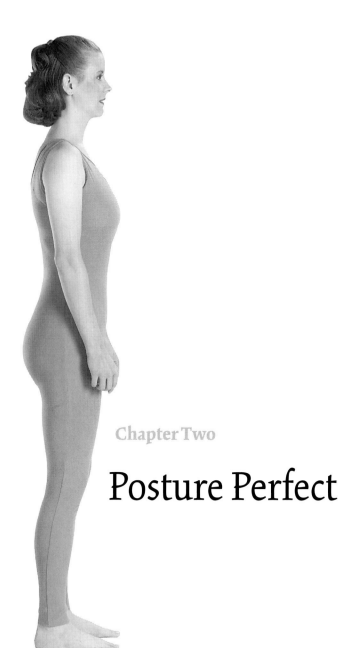

Chapter Two

Posture Perfect

"STAND UP STRAIGHT, DON'T SLOUCH." "Stomach in, chest out, shoulders down." "Tuck your tailbone under." "Don't tuck your tailbone." "Bend your knees." "Pull your shoulders back." These are just some of the admonitions we've heard about posture. But none answers the basic question, What should I do to improve my alignment?

Alignment is one of the most important—and most misunderstood—concepts in fitness. Different exercise systems offer conflicting advice on body placement. It's no surprise that many of us have a misguided idea of what good posture is. To complicate matters, most of our postural habits are unconscious. Poor posture feels natural and comfortable. Primary movement patterns are set in early childhood and typically mimic those of one or both parents. As we get older, we begin to emulate what we see in society and often adopt the postures of those we admire.

Women are at a particular disadvantage. Why? Because almost every female image in magazines, on TV, and (most unforgivably) in fitness publications has a hyperextended pelvis and/or spine. The look is so universal that most of us don't even notice it. It is considered attractive and desirable.

When the spine is balanced in the upright neutral position, weight support is achieved primarily through the bones. Some intermittent work is done by the long muscles of the back and by the abdominals to maintain the spine's equilibrium. The benefits of a neutral spine are numerous:

- improved body mechanics and neuromuscular efficiency
- improved body contours and a more slender appearance
- reduction and/or elimination of pain
- prevention of injury
- slowed aging process
- increased flexibility
- increased blood flow
- improved sense of balance and coordination
- better sleeping patterns
- ease of emotional issues that have been held in the body
- improved quality of life.

The body is in the upright neutral position when its various parts are symmetrically aligned around the line of gravity that runs through it. When viewed from the side, the line of gravity bisects the head at the level of the ear, the middle of the thorax, hip sockets, and knees, and slightly in front of the ankle joints. The spine displays its signature "S" curve. When viewed from the front, the line of gravity divides the body into right and left sides. Ideally, both hip sockets and shoulder tips will be on the same horizontal plane. **(2b)**

The weight of pregnancy changes the body's center of gravity, and in turn the spine realigns to find a new state of equilibrium. When misaligned, the body must work harder to maintain the upright position. Muscle groups that are not designed for postural support get called on to take up some of the slack. Through habitual overuse, these muscles become overly tight, or hypertonic, and sometimes spasm painfully. Hypertonic muscles place mechanical strain on the joints, cartilage, ligaments, and tendons (which connect muscle to bone). This greatly increases the likelihood of wear-and-tear injuries and osteoarthritis. Hypertonic muscles also decrease the body's range of motion.

To relieve tired and hypertonic muscles, the body sags into the ligaments, compressing the intervertebral discs, veins, and soft tissues, decreasing blood flow. This increases the discomfort and healing time of common postpartum conditions such as hemorrhoids, episiotomy stitches, perineum tearing,

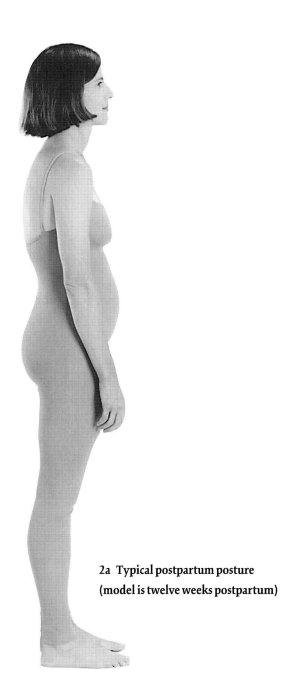

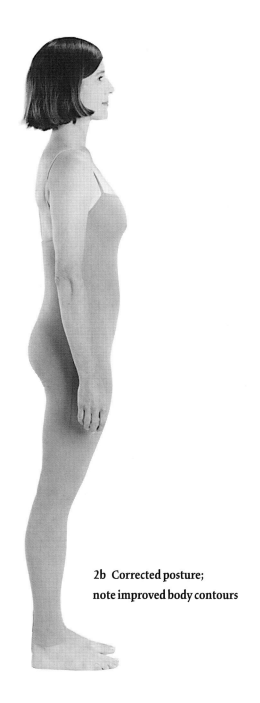

2a Typical postpartum posture
(model is twelve weeks postpartum)

2b Corrected posture;
note improved body contours

vulval edema, and cesarean recovery. **(2a)**

Of course, perfect posture is a concept. No one has a symmetrical body. Many of us have minor structural anomalies, such as rolled arches or knock knees, that alter alignment. And since we are moving all the time, good posture is not a static position we must hold rigidly. What we're going for is functional balance.

The Pelvis (2-1)

Good alignment depends on the pelvis. A neutral spine can be developed only when its base, the pelvis, is in the neutral position. The pelvis is often described as bowl-shaped. And it is, but it's a bowl with very little front and no bottom. Three pairs of bones make up the pelvis, and each pair has right and left sides. The largest bone, the ilium, forms the sides and back of the pelvis. This bone is felt when we put our hands on our hips. At the center back the ilium connects with the sacral vertebrae at the sacroiliac joint. The ligaments of the sacroiliac joint are very dense. Most people have limited movement, if any, at this joint, though some gliding motion is possible. Many women feel pain in the sacroiliac joint after pregnancy due to ligament laxity. If you are experiencing instability or pain in this joint, you should avoid movements that stretch the back of the pelvis, such as sitting with your legs crossed, stretching in the tailor position, or doing any of the Lotus-type yoga poses.

The pubic bones make up the front rim of the pelvis. They are fused together at the front of the pelvis, the pubic symphasis. This joint normally has no movement. During pregnancy, however, the hormones that soften and elongate the ligaments allow the pubic symphasis to separate slightly to accommodate the baby's passage through the bottom of the pelvis. Sometimes women feel pain at this joint after pregnancy. Like women who experience pain in the sacroiliac, you want to avoid positions that stress this joint, such as straddle stretches. Use pain as your guide.

If it hurts, don't do it; don't try to stretch through the pain.

The third bone of the pelvis, the ischium, often referred to as the sits bone, is at the bottom. It's the bone you can rock back and forth on when you're sitting on the floor.

The pelvis bones are fused together and connected to the sacral vertebrae, which are also fused. Because these are fused joints, the pelvis always moves as a unit. It is the body's hub and literal center of gravity, with the spine and lower limbs radiating outward.

The inclination of the pelvis has a direct effect on the spine and an indirect effect on the placement of most bones in the body. An anterior tilt of the pelvis, also known as a lordotic posture, sends the tailbone back and increases the curve of the lower (lumbar) spine. **(2-1b)**

A posterior tilt, or kyphotic posture, tucks the tailbone under, moves the pubic bone forward, and flattens the lumbar curve of the spine. The kyphotic posture increases the curve of the upper back, or thorax. In response, the head glides down and forward. **(2-1c)** Thanks to the prevalence of computers and a sedentary lifestyle, the kyphotic posture is now the most common postural misalignment in our society.

After pregnancy, we find ourselves with a combination lordotic-kyphotic posture: a tipped pelvis, too much curve in the lower spine, too much curve in the upper spine, and a forward head.

These postural patterns tend to be self-reinforcing. Overly tight muscles are a result of poor posture and continue to pull the bones out of alignment. Opposing muscle groups are underused and atrophy and weaken, further reinforcing the pattern. After pregnancy, women lack functional use of the abdominal wall, and cannot stabilize the pelvis and lower back.

Though these body systems are complex, there is a simple way to find the neutral position in your pelvis: identification of what I call the bikini triangle.

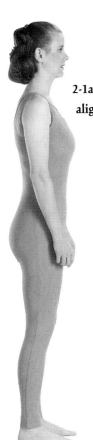

2-1a Ideal neutral alignment

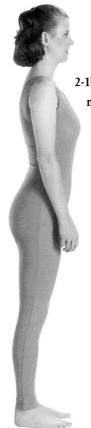

2-1b Lordotic posture; note anterior tilt of the pelvis (tailbone back)

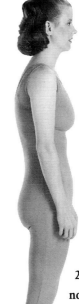

2-1c Kyphotic posture: note posterior tilt of the pelvis (tailbone tucked) with overly curved upper back and forward head

The Bikini Triangle (2-2)

To find your bikini triangle, stand and place your hands on the front of your hips. The bony prominence you feel is the anterior crest of the ilium. Place the heels of your hands on your ilium, and point your fingers diagonally toward your groin. At the midline of your body you will feel your pubic bone. Imagine a line that runs through these three points. This is your bikini triangle.

When you stand in the neutral position your bikini triangle is vertical and parallel to the wall in front of you. Ideally, the anterior crests of the ilium are the same distance from the floor. Try to identify this position while standing in front of a mirror. **(2-2a)** Sometimes it's easier to see if you stand at a slight diagonal rather than facing the mirror straight on. **(2-2b)** Note the position of your bones. Identify the natural "S" curve of your spine. Some spines are fairly flat, while others are more curvaceous.

Adjust your pubic bone either forward or back so that your bikini triangle is vertical. Lengthen your spine, pulling your body weight out of your lower back. Allow your shoulders to drop. Evaluate your head position. A forward head is almost universal after pregnancy. Push the back of your head up and back to align your ears over your shoulders. Your chin will naturally rotate slightly toward your chest. Take a look at yourself now; not only will you look trimmer and healthier, you'll also feel better.

Many of the exercises in this book start with the body in the neutral supine position, sometimes called the "hook lying position" **(see p. 24).** When you're in this position, your bikini triangle will be flat, parallel to the floor, and on the tabletop, or transverse, plane. In all of the exercises, you will be asked to move or stabilize your pelvis and hence your bikini triangle. This precision and control is the foundation of dynamic stability exercises and is critical to establishing good movement patterns and developing core strength.

Identifying your bikini triangle is fairly easy, but stabilizing it during movement is not—especially after pregnancy. Your abdominal muscles have lost tone and strength. You may feel as if your pelvic area and abdominal muscles are lost in a fog in the first postpartum weeks. Stabilizing your spine may seem impossible. How can you contract a muscle you can't find?

Mental imagery can make a world of difference. A clear mental picture of the desired movement helps the nervous system choose the most efficient movement pathway. Soon your muscles will begin to kick in. Repetition of the desired movement with a clear mental focus is the fastest way to teach your body new skills. And in terms of pelvic stability, practice will make perfect, sooner than you think.

2-2a
Bikini triangle,
front view

2-2b
Bikini triangle,
diagonal view

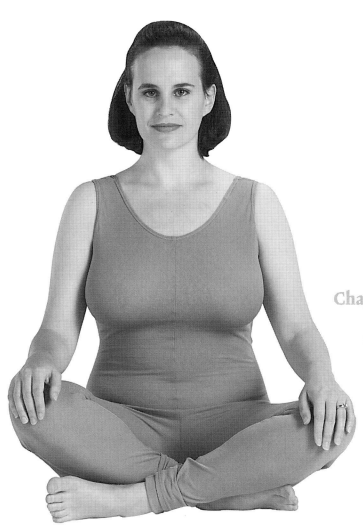

Chapter Three

The Pelvic Floor

Several months after the birth of my son, I was sitting in my kitchen when I suddenly sneezed. Like a car airbag, my pelvic floor exploded into the chair with a force that shocked me. I had thought I knew what postpartum laxity was all about. I had thought I was almost finished retoning my pelvic floor. That sneeze told me otherwise.

The muscles of the pelvic floor can get blown away by a vaginal birth. And though the area is rather small, its importance is huge. The pelvic floor muscles have attachments at the pubic bone in front, the tailbone, or coccyx, at the rear, and laterally at the ischium (the bottom bones of the pelvis). Viewed from below, these bony landmarks form a slightly flattened diamond. Take a moment to identify these bones in your body.

The pelvic floor muscles have four basic functions:

- support for the pelvic organs and their contents

- urinary and bowel sphincter control

- support during increases of intra-abdominal pressure caused by bodily functions such as laughing, coughing, and sneezing, as well as by physical exertion such as crunches, jumping, and lifting heavy objects

- reproductive and sexual activities.

Like the abdominals, the pelvic floor muscles don't automatically regain their former length or tone. They must be reconditioned so that good functional control can be reestablished. And it is essential that you reestablish tone in the pelvic floor before jumping into traditional abdominal exercises such as crunches and reverse curls. During these types of exercises intra-abdominal pressure increases dramatically, especially if you hold your breath. If the pelvic floor is not strong enough, it will balloon out. Pushing down through the pelvic floor puts strain on episiotomy stitches or tearing, exacerbates hemorrhoid problems, and negates the benefits of Kegel exercises.

The pelvic floor muscles have both voluntary and involuntary muscle fibers. As part of the involuntary system, a mild state of contraction provides bladder and bowel control. Embedded in the pelvic floor are two circular sphincter muscles that resemble a figure eight. The frontal opening encompasses the urethra and vagina, with the rectum at the rear. Between the sphincters is a strong band of connective tissue called the perineum. This area is cut during an episiotomy. The second important muscle group is the levator ani, which, as its name suggests, lifts the pelvic floor into the abdominal cavity. After pregnancy and childbirth, the pelvic floor muscles sag and become hammock-shaped, rather than flat across. Simply contracting the sphincter muscles during Kegels is not enough. You must also learn to voluntarily contract the levator ani group, and shorten its fibers, to reestablish adequate support for the internal organs.

Reconditioning the pelvic floor is not just for those who have had a vaginal delivery. Many women have a cesarean delivery after hours of pushing, resulting in at least a partially stretched pelvic floor. And even with a planned cesarean, the weight of the baby in late pregnancy can stretch and weaken the pelvic floor.

A lax pelvic floor can cause several problems. The most common after childbirth is urinary stress incontinence, the involuntary release of urine when laughing, coughing, sneezing, running, etc. If left untreated, the problem can worsen with subsequent pregnancies, weight gain, and aging. Women who do not adequately retone the pelvic floor may have problems for years. A more serious problem, uterine and/or bladder prolapse, occurs when the organs sag onto the vagina. This condition often requires surgery to correct.

Hopefully, your doctor or midwife introduced you to Kegel exercises while you were pregnant. They are easier to learn before your tissues stretch. If not, don't worry. Here is a terrific pelvic floor conditioner—one that strengthens both the levator ani group and the sphincters.

Super Kegels

❶ Sit on a hard chair or the floor. Stretch your spine toward the ceiling.

❷ Exhale, imagine that you need to stop a bowel movement, and squeeze your anal sphincter closed. Take a normal breath as you maintain closure of your anus.

❸ Exhale, imagine that you need to stop the flow of urine, and close your vaginal sphincter. Take a normal breath as you maintain the closure of both sphincters. (Some women find it helpful to imagine that they are squeezing their labia together to more deeply activate their vaginal sphincter.)

❹ Exhale, imagine that you are pulling your tailbone and pubic bone toward the center of your pelvic floor. Visualize laces between the two bones that you pull taut. This will contract the levator ani group. Hold the contraction for three seconds.

❺ Exhale and relax. Notice how your pelvic floor softens and widens.

❻ Pelvic floor reconditioning can be started a day or two after childbirth. At first you won't be able to feel much of anything, but with regular practice your muscles will be-

gin to respond. Many women complain that only the anal sphincter seems to be contracting. Sometimes it takes a while for the vaginal sphincter to get with the program, especially if you had a long pushing phase during childbirth. And Mother Nature is no fool: the anal sphincter is naturally the much stronger of the two.

Pelvic floor exercises help ease pain from perineum tears, episiotomy stitches, vulval edema, and hemorrhoids. When the sphincters contract, the tissues are pushed closer together, decreasing pressure. The increased blood flow to the area helps speed healing. Strong pelvic floor muscles also enhance sexual pleasure for you and your partner.

Mental imagery is particularly useful for these exercises. Feel free to make up your own visualizations. Breathe normally through the contractions. If you find it difficult to breathe, you are probably contracting your diaphragm and/or tightening your abdominal muscles. Relax the area around your rib cage and belly and try again.

If you find that the large muscles of your butt (the gluteals) are contracting, try practicing the contractions in positions where your hips are deeply flexed, such as squatting, or lying on your back with your legs pulled toward your chest.

Don't practice Kegels with your legs crossed. This is not an effective position to isolate the pelvic floor. You will feel a lot of groin action, but you will primarily be using your inner thighs, not your pelvic floor.

After you get good at contracting your pelvic floor muscles, you can do Kegels almost anywhere, any time. If you have hemorrhoids or have stretched your anal sphincter, it is particularly helpful to do a set after you have a bowel movement.

Since the pelvic floor muscles fatigue easily, do a small number of them at a time. Start with five or six repetitions per set and repeat the sets many times throughout the day. You are going for volume here. Plan on doing ten to twelve (or even more) sets a day.

How do you know when you've sufficiently toned your pelvic floor? When you can stop a full stream of urine without any leakage. However, stopping urine should only be used as a test. Do not practice pelvic floor contractions during urination, as it can interfere with emptying the bladder completely, which in turn can cause urinary tract infections.

Finding the pelvic floor muscles and contracting them after childbirth can be a challenge. Don't give up. Keep trying and maintain mental focus, even if you think nothing much is happening. As your muscle fibers shorten and you gain neuromuscular efficiency, you will be able to recruit a deeper response. Depending on your level of physical conditioning, the type of labor you had, and number of sets you do, reconditioning the pelvic floor can take anywhere from six weeks to six months.

Chapter Four

The Abdominal Wall

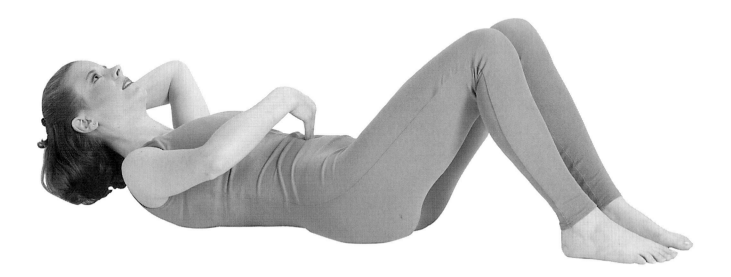

T HE MOST OBVIOUS and often most distressing aspect of having a postpartum body is the extreme laxity of the abdominal wall. By the end of pregnancy, the abdominal muscles have been stretched to near maximum potential. After childbirth, the tissue is extremely lax and soft. This takes a lot of first-time mothers by surprise. I know it surprised me. As a dancer and fitness trainer, I was stunned that muscle tissue could be so spongy—what I like to call the "pudding effect."

The uterus, stimulated by breast-feeding, continues to contract after childbirth and automatically returns to close to its former size in a matter of weeks. The abdominal muscles aren't so lucky. Like the pelvic floor, they must be reconditioned. But because of several postpartum factors, reconditioning must be systematic to avoid complications and hasten recovery.

The abdominal wall is comprised of four main muscle groups; each has a right and left side. They all share a band of connective tissue at the midline of the body, the linea alba. During pregnancy this area often darkens and is referred to as the linea negra.

THE ABDOMINAL RECTUS

The abdominal rectus muscle, the most exterior layer of the four, runs vertically from the lower ribs to the pubic bone. Perhaps the most easily recognized of the abdominals, in well-conditioned men it is sometimes referred to as a "six pack." The rectus is responsible for spine flexion—moving the rib cage and pelvic bones closer together. It is developed with crunches and reverse curls.

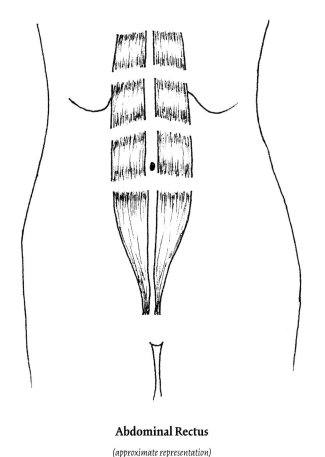

Abdominal Rectus

(approximate representation)

Abdominal Separation

In some women, pregnancy causes abdominal separation, in which the two sides of the abdominal rectus separate at the body's midline. You can think of it like a zipper that pops open in the middle. It can appear any time after the second trimester of pregnancy and reaches its peak as the uterus expands to its full size. For some women the condition does not resolve after childbirth. The gap can occur above, below, or, most commonly, at the level of the belly button. Abdominal separation in one pregnancy greatly increases the likelihood of the condition in later pregnancies. It reduces the integrity of the abdominal wall and can aggravate lower back pain.

It is imperative to know whether you have this condition before you resume abdominal exercises. Certain exercises create shear forces that can pull the separation farther apart and must be avoided until the condition has resolved. Other specific postpartum exercises work to close the gap and train the rectus to realign at the midline.

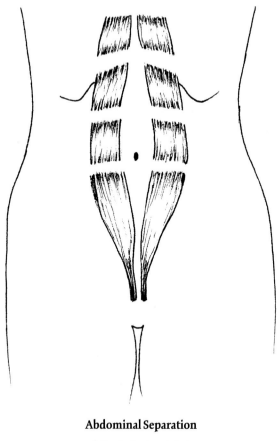

Abdominal Separation

(approximate representation)

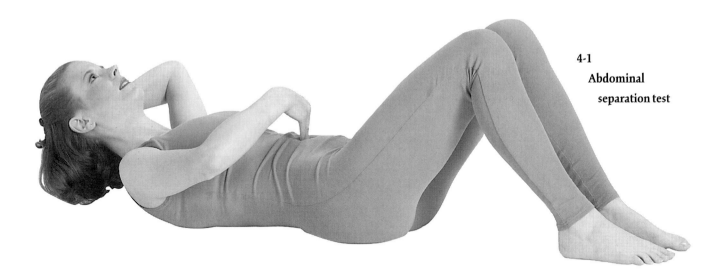

4-1
Abdominal
separation test

Test for Abdominal Separation (4-1)

❶ Lie on your back, knees bent and feet flat on the floor.

❷ Place one hand behind your head for support, and put your other hand on your belly, fingers across the midline. (The palm of that hand will point toward your face.) Push your fingers into your belly. After pregnancy, it is common to feel a bottomless pit at your belly button.

❸ Lift your head and shoulders slightly off the floor as you contract your abdominals. You will be able to feel the parallel bands of your abdominal rectus muscle.

❹ Test at the level of your belly button as well as above and below. The more fingers you can fit into the gap, the more severe the separation.

If you are less than six weeks postpartum, it is normal to have a small gap, two fingers wide or less. If your gap is more than two fingers wide, regardless of how postpartum you are, you need to do abdominal splinting exercises—no traditional crunches—until the gap is two fingers or less or until your connective tissue has shortened. In this case, the gap, though still wider than two fingers, will be extremely shallow with a strong, elastic base.

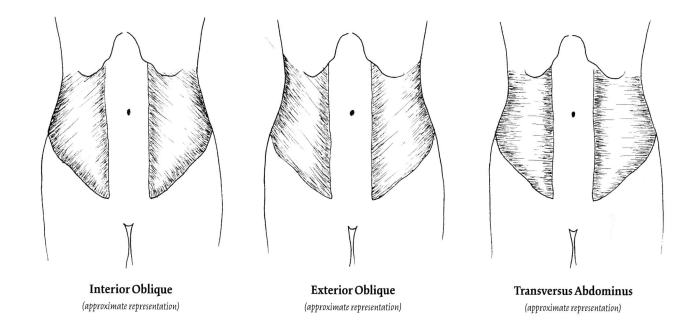

Interior Oblique
(approximate representation)

Exterior Oblique
(approximate representation)

Transversus Abdominus
(approximate representation)

THE EXTERIOR AND INTERIOR OBLIQUES

The exterior and interior oblique muscles run in contrasting diagonals across the front of the body. They connect to the lower ribs and attach to the pelvis. The obliques flex the spine to the side and help rotate the spine around its central axis. Most importantly, they wrap around the back and insert into the lumbar fascia (connective tissue) of the lower back. Because they have insertions at both the front midline and the lower back, the obliques play a critical but often overlooked role in alignment and stabilization of the lumbar vertebrae. After pregnancy, reconditioning the obliques helps flatten the abdominal wall and redefine the waistline.

THE TRANSVERSUS ABDOMINUS

The transversus abdominus, the deepest layer of the abdominal wall, has fibers that run horizontally across the abdomen and is commonly referred to as the "waist cincher" muscle. When contracted, the transversus compresses the abdomen. Its fibers wrap front to back, have insertions at the lower ribs and the pelvis, and, like the obliques, connect to the lumbar fascia. Working with the obliques, the transversus supports the internal organs and stabilizes the pelvis and lower spine.

The transversus plays a crucial role in reconditioning after pregnancy. Contraction of the transversus compresses and flattens the abdominal wall and draws the belly toward the spine. This action also pulls the abdominal rectus toward the body's midline, which helps to internally close abdominal separation. In addition, contraction of the transversus before a crunch or other abdominal work helps contain intra-abdominal pressure so that the belly doesn't bulge on exertion. **(5-6b, p. 30)**

Interestingly, the transversus does not automatically contract with the obliques and the rectus. During a traditional crunch the obliques and the rectus always work together; it is impossible to isolate one from the other. However, if the transversus is not consciously contracted, it will not join in. This has important implications for all types of abdominal conditioning exercises.

Many of the exercises in Chapter Six help you find and strengthen your transversus. For many women, this will be a new experience. Even if you are no longer postpartum, it is critical that you don't skip or skim over the initial exercises. Take time to learn them. The first group of exercises prepares you for the more advanced work.

The Pyramidalis

The pyramidalis, the smallest of the abdominal muscles, can be absent in some individuals. This triangular muscle has its apex at the belly button and fans out to connect to the pubic bone. When contracted, the pyramidalis lifts and stabilizes the front of the pelvis. As with the transversus, it must be consciously contracted. This is a difficult muscle to find, especially postpartum, but you can feel its action during a cough, sneeze, or laughter.

Muscle Functions

During movement, any given muscle group may have one of four functions. Muscle groups that contract concentrically to produce movement function as prime movers, or agonists. Working in opposition to agonists, antagonists lengthen, or eccentrically contract, to allow movement to occur. For example, when the knee is straightened, the muscles on the front of the thigh, the quadriceps, contract concentrically and function as prime movers. Simultaneously the back of the thigh, the hamstrings, lengthen and function as antagonists. Muscle groups that assist prime movers function as secondary movers. Muscle groups that maintain body positioning function as stabilizers and contract isometrically; in this case, muscle length remains the same and therefore no movement occurs. For example, during a standing biceps curl, the muscles of the torso contract isometrically so that the body remains stable and upright during the exercise.

When functioning as prime movers, the abdominals flex the spine to the front and sides, and help rotate the spine around its central axis. In addition, the abdominals (particularly the obliques and transversus) stabilize the pelvis and spine. The abdominals must be trained to function as both prime movers and stabilizers. In many people, whether they've had a baby or not, lack of stabilization is a primary cause of lower back pain and many wear-and-tear injuries of the spine.

Chapter Five

Getting Started

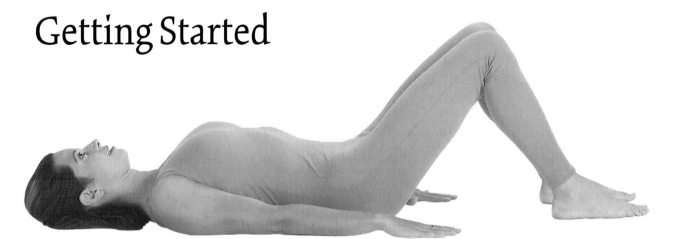

Because alignment is crucial for good neuromuscular technique, how you prepare your body for exercise greatly influences the benefits it provides. When you start in a properly aligned and stabilized position, it is easier to maintain good form during exercise. You get the most of each repetition. Good form coupled with mental focus is the most effective way to achieve fitness goals.

Many of the following exercises ask you to prepare your body in a specific position. Familiarize yourself with the following positions to maximize the benefits of your sessions.

Neutral Supine Position (5-1)

❶ Lie on your back, legs bent, soles of your feet on the floor, arms by your side. There should be a gap of four or five inches between your knees and between your ankles. Make sure that your toes face forward. (This is a much narrower position than that used in many sports techniques.) There should be about eighteen inches between your heels and your hips. Your legs are now aligned in first position parallel.

❷ Your pelvis should be neutral, with your bikini triangle parallel to the floor. Try rocking your pelvis by pushing gently through the legs to release excess muscle tension. When neutral, your pubic bone lies flat between your legs and your lumbar curve (waist) is off the floor. Many of us automatically flatten our lumbar curve when we lie down.

Place your hands on your bikini triangle to feel whether your pelvis is neutral.

❸ The shoulders are neutral as well. Roll slightly to your left side so that your body weight comes off your right shoulder blade; pull your shoulder blade an inch or so down your back. Take care that you do not accidentally move your rib cage. Rock to the other side and pull your other shoulder down. Return to center. Both shoulder blades are now well down the back. Your shoulder tips should be closer to the floor and farther from your ears. Allow the back of your rib cage to relax on the floor.

❹ To align your head, lengthen your neck by rotating the back of your head away from your torso; your chin will rotate toward your chest. Keep your head on the floor. If you are very tight in the upper shoulders or have a pronounced forward head posture, you may be more comfortable with a small paperback book behind your head. Depending on your size, an inch to inch-and-one-half lift is appropriate. Don't use a pillow, as they tend to flex the front of the neck and increase forward head problems.

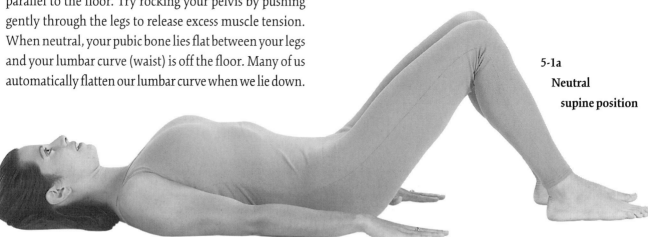

5-1a
Neutral
supine position

Exercise After Pregnancy: How to Look and Feel Your Best

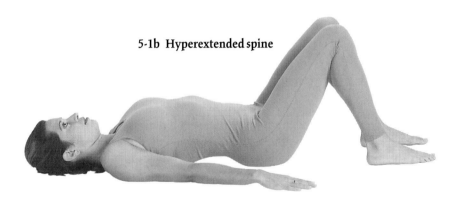

5-1b Hyperextended spine

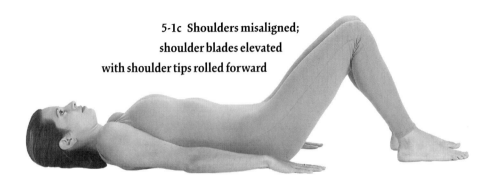

5-1c Shoulders misaligned;
shoulder blades elevated
with shoulder tips rolled forward

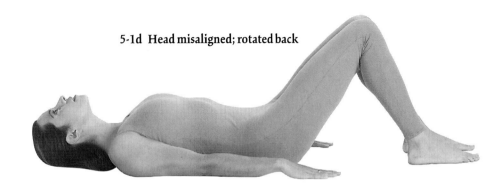

5-1d Head misaligned; rotated back

Hollow Pelvic Tilt Position (5-2)

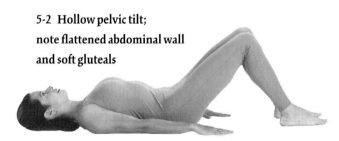

5-2 Hollow pelvic tilt;
note flattened abdominal wall
and soft gluteals

❶ Start in the neutral supine position. Tighten your abdominal wall.

❷ Deepen the pull of your abdominal wall as you curl your tailbone toward the ceiling. Strongly pull your belly button toward your spine. Your bikini triangle is now on a tilt. Take care that your gluteals (butt) stay soft. Try not to press into the floor with your legs and feet. Your muscular effort should be focused between your pubic bone and belly button. Keep your rib cage and shoulders relaxed. Breathe normally.

Hollow Tuck Position (5-3)

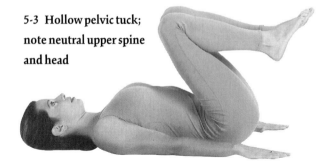

5-3 Hollow pelvic tuck;
note neutral upper spine
and head

❶ Start in the neutral supine position. Tighten your abdominal wall and anchor your lumbar spine to the floor with a hollow pelvic tilt.

❷ Without wobbling, bring your right knee up toward your chest. Bring your left knee up beside it. Allow your lower limbs and feet to relax. Press your shoulder tips lightly toward the floor, keeping the back of your neck long.

❸ Close your pelvic floor. Pull your abdominal wall down toward your spine as much as you can. Visualize a zipper that runs from your tailbone to your pubic bone and from your pubic bone to your sternum; pull it closed tight.

❹ Pull both knees as close to your chest as possible. (Use your lower abdominals and hip flexors, not your hands.) Make sure your thighs and lower legs are parallel to each other.

Quadruped Position (5-4)

❶ Get on all fours. Align your thighs and arms so they are perpendicular to the floor. If you have pain in your wrists, make fists and support your arms on the fists, keeping your wrists neutral.

❷ Move your pubic bone so that your bikini triangle is parallel to the floor. Strongly pull your belly away from the floor to support your pelvis and lumbar spine. Don't try to make a flat back.

❸ Pull your shoulder blades down your back and slightly together. Push firmly away from the floor with your arms. Take care that this does not round your upper spine.

❹ Lengthen the back of your neck, rotating your chin toward your chest.

Many of us have been conditioned to tuck the tailbone under or push through the spine to flatten the lumbar curve. If you can, try this position in front of a mirror. You want to find and support a neutral spine. When you are in a good quadruped position you will feel very powerful, like a carnivore. If you allow your spine to sag, shoulders to hunch, or head to drop, you will feel weak, more like a grazing herbivore.

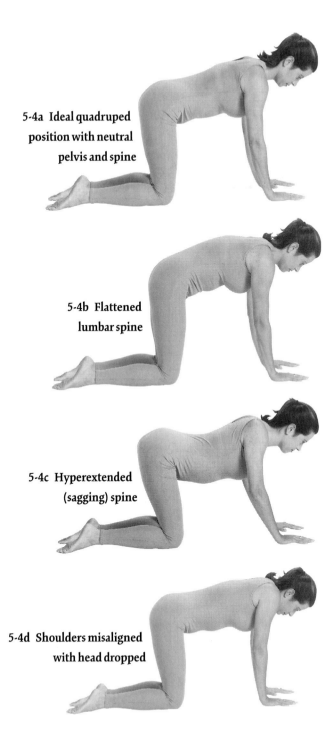

5-4a Ideal quadruped position with neutral pelvis and spine

5-4b Flattened lumbar spine

5-4c Hyperextended (sagging) spine

5-4d Shoulders misaligned with head dropped

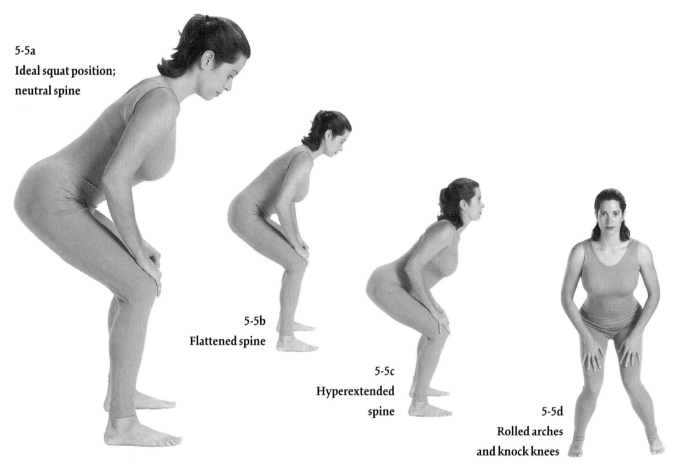

5-5a
Ideal squat position;
neutral spine

5-5b
Flattened spine

5-5c
Hyperextended
spine

5-5d
Rolled arches
and knock knees

Squat Position (5-5)

❶ Stand with your pelvis neutral and your feet slightly wider than your hips, knees and feet facing forward. This is second position parallel.

❷ Tighten your abdominal wall. Lengthen your spine upward, pulling your body weight out of your lower back. Push your shoulder blades down your back and slightly together. Lengthen the back of your neck; align your ears over your shoulders.

❸ Simultaneously bend at the hips, knees, and ankles. Your pelvis and spine will move as a unit from vertical to a high diagonal. The curves of your spine do not change. Keep your knees aligned over your toes, the arches of your feet intact. Evenly distribute your body weight between your heels and the balls of your feet. **(5-5a)**

❹ Lower the squat by deepening the bend of your hips, knees, and ankles. Keep your abdominal wall tight. Go only as low as you can maintain a neutral spine.

Exercise After Pregnancy: How to Look and Feel Your Best

Abdominal Wall
Training Techniques (5-6)

Abdominal exercises can be a pain in the neck, literally. Neck pain during crunches is a very common problem. It can occur at the front or the back, or sometimes in both places. Many people have a tendency to overwork their arms, shoulders, and chest (none of which, of course, are abdominal muscles) during crunches. This occurs as compensation for weak abdominal muscles or in an overzealous attempt to tone the area. I will discuss some of these problems in detail and offer solutions.

Pain in the front of the neck occurs when your head is overly flexed at the beginning of a crunch, especially if you've been taught to roll your head off the floor before lifting your shoulders. Sometimes your head overflexes near the end of the movement when you try to go deeper into the crunch. **(5-6c)** Instead of using more abdominal muscle, you pull through your head and neck. Remember, the muscles of your abdominal wall connect to your lower ribs. This is where you want to initiate the movement. Ideally, your neck muscles stabilize your head and neck during a crunch. **(5-6a)**

The standing crunch is a good test of your abdominal technique. Stand in front of a mirror with both knees bent and your hands behind your head; mimic a crunch by tightening your abdominals and pulling your rib cage closer to your hips. The distance between your chin and chest should not change. Keep your chest and shoulder muscles relaxed; the distance between your elbows should not change, and of course you should not yank on your head. Your head and neck just go along for the ride.

Your may find it helpful to place a small ball between your chin and chest during crunches. As you roll up, take care not to squeeze the ball with your chin. A baby's squeak toy works great because if you overflex your head, the toy will make noise. You can use a rolled-up pair of socks if you don't have the right size toy. Another technique for stabilizing your head is to press your tongue to the roof of your mouth as you work. This will contract the internal muscles of the neck, aiding stabilization.

If you tend to yank your body off the floor with your arms, focus on relaxing your shoulders, chest, and arms. Allow your head to rest in your hands. Concentrate on moving your rib cage toward your pelvis. Your shoulders won't go up as high off the floor, but your positioning will be greatly improved and you will use your abdominals more effectively.

Pain in the back of the neck is associated with the head rotating back during the roll-down phase of a crunch and/or a starting alignment in which the head is rotated back (the chin points to the ceiling). **(5-6d)** This position is common for people with a forward head or kyphotic posture. Strongly rotate your chin to your chest so that your neck lengthens and the back of your head rests farther away from your torso. Try to maintain the length of the back of your neck and the rotation of your head as you work your abdominals. A ball is also helpful because if you rotate your head back, you will drop the ball.

Another common problem associated with posterior neck pain is what I call the "chicken." **(5-6e)** Many people become very conscious of not overflexing their necks during abdominal work. But at the last moment, they try too hard to get higher off the floor and push their heads toward the ceiling in a birdlike pulse. This action compresses the back of the skull

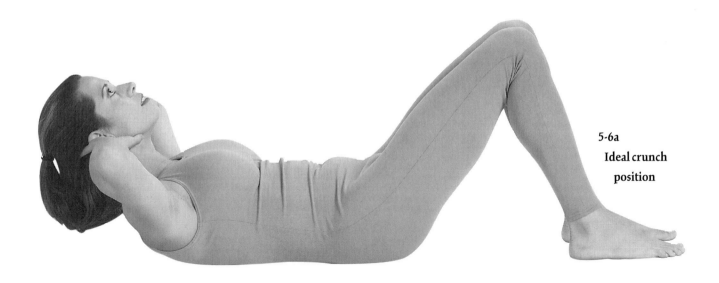

5-6a
Ideal crunch
position

onto the cervical vertebrae, causing pain. If you have this problem, focus your energy below your rib cage. Allow your head and neck to simply go along for the ride.

Perhaps the most common misalignment during abdominal training is hyperextension of the shoulder blades as the hands reach up to support the back of the head and neck. This is prevalent after childbirth because the muscles on the tops of the shoulders are overly tight. Make sure that you start with your shoulder blades well down your back, and keep them there as you put your hands behind your head. See Chapter Seven for more details about crunches.

Some individuals, particularly those who work with computers, hyperextend their wrists as they prepare for abdominal work. **(5-6f)** This can be particularly dangerous after pregnancy, when the body is more vulnerable to carpal tunnel syndrome and other repetitive stress injuries. If you have this tendency or have any wrist problems or pain, no matter how minor, use the fists variation. Make fists. Align your

wrists so that they are neutral. Place your fists behind your ears, putting your knuckles in contact with your head. **(5-6g)** Though this position offers less stability and support to the head and neck, it is safe for the wrists. And because it provides less support, your crunches may be a little smaller, especially in the beginning. See Chapter Nine for more details about carpal tunnel syndrome.

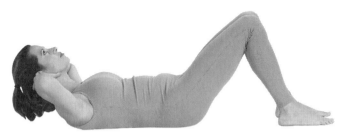

5-6b Abdomen protruding during a crunch

Exercise After Pregnancy: How to Look and Feel Your Best

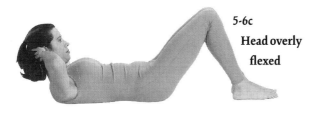

5-6c
**Head overly
flexed**

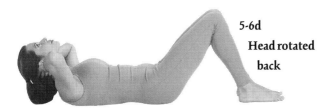

5-6d
**Head rotated
back**

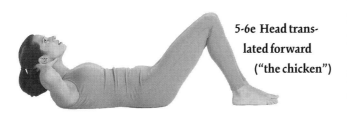

5-6e **Head trans-
lated forward
("the chicken")**

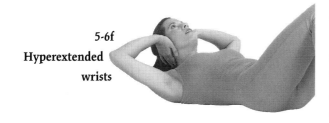

5-6f
**Hyperextended
wrists**

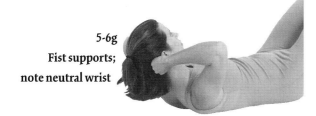

5-6g
**Fist supports;
note neutral wrist**

How To Use This Book

Plan on learning the exercises in the order given. Work slowly through them so that you understand what you're trying to achieve. When you start a chapter, you may only perform five or six exercises in a session. As you become more familiar with the program, you can add exercises until you can perform a full workout in one session. The postpartum workout in Chapter Six can be performed in about twenty minutes when you know the exercises well. The subsequent workouts in Chapters Seven and Eight should take about forty minutes to complete.

Once you're familiar with the exercises, feel free to adapt them to your needs. For instance, if you are experiencing a lot of upper back pain and fatigue, the Spiral Stretch, Shoulder Stretch, and Neck Stretch can help realign your upper body, release overly tight muscles, and relieve pain.

Because new mothers have so little free time, don't try to box yourself in with an overly demanding workout schedule. If your baby takes short, sporadic naps, plan on breaking an exercise session into two or three segments throughout the day. If your baby takes long naps (lucky you!), you can complete a workout in one session.

The postpartum exercises are gentle enough to perform every day. Depending on your physical conditioning, you may experience some muscle soreness after practicing the exercises in Chapter Seven. If you do, take a rest day between your workouts. Most women will need a rest day between the workouts in Chapter Eight.

For those who simply want to be fit enough for the tasks of daily life or need to return to work soon after childbirth, the exercises in Chapter Seven are designed to meet those goals. Don't feel bad if you don't make it through the advanced workout in Chapter Eight. It is aimed at those who want to achieve a very high level of fitness.

Chapter Six

Step 1: Postpartum Exercises

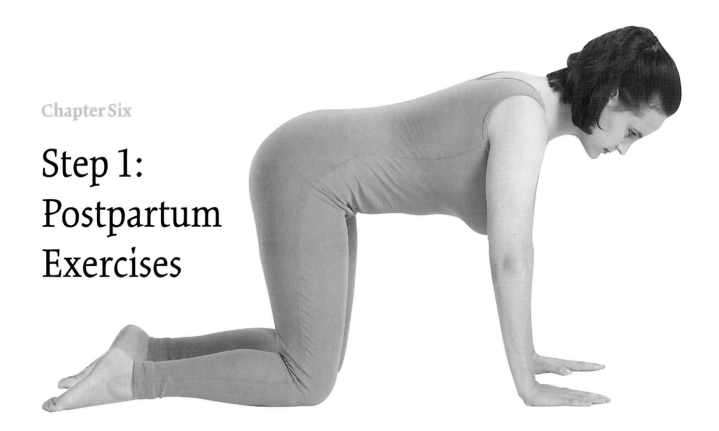

UNLIKE MOST EXERCISE PROGRAMS, which are designed to challenge the body, postpartum exercises are gentle and nonstressful. They are designed to hasten the recovery from childbirth, reduce pain and discomfort, and establish the basic physical skills that the more demanding exercises in this book build upon.

As you learn the following exercises, work slowly and carefully. Monitor your body. None of the exercises should hurt or cause strain. Stay within your personal comfort zone. Focus on the quality of your actions and where your body is in space rather than on how many repetitions you can do.

These exercises can be started any time after childbirth—whenever you feel ready to begin rebuilding your body. Practice them until you are four to six weeks postpartum and your lochia (the bleeding after childbirth) has stopped. If you had a cesarean delivery or major tearing, wait until your stitches have completely healed before you begin postpartum exercises.

If you are beginning the exercise program and are more than six weeks postpartum, plan on spending at least several weeks learning these exercises to prepare your body for the more challenging exercises in Chapter Seven. I have seen many women at six or even nine months postpartum who still need to establish the foundations of good body usage—neutral alignment, functional core strength, and dynamic stability. After pregnancy, everyone needs to start with the basics.

Discontinue the exercises immediately and consult your doctor if your lochia suddenly increases and/or turns bright red; you develop a fever, infection, or mastitis (inflammation of the mammary glands); or you feel sharp pain or severe discomfort anywhere in your body.

Belly Lacing (6-1)

❶ Lie on your right side, spine long, knees bent, right arm bent under your head for support. (You can use a small pillow instead of your arm.) Relax your belly, allowing it to expand and fall to the floor. **(6-1a)**

❷ Place your left hand across the lowest part of your belly, just above your pubic bone. Strongly contract your pelvic floor muscles. Take a normal breath. On the next exhale, imagine that you are lacing up an old-fashioned corset as you pull your belly off the floor and in toward your spine. Use your hand to help lift and "lace" your belly closed at your midline. Try not to move your spine. Keep your shoulders relaxed. Hold your belly in as you take a normal breath. **(6-1b)**

❸ Place your left hand slightly higher on your lower abdomen. On the next exhale, pull your belly farther off the floor and into your spine as you press your belly up and in with your hand. Take a normal breath, maintaining the tightness of your abdominal wall.

❹ Repeat the lacing two more times as you work your way up to your rib cage.

❺ On the last sequence, put your left hand across your lowest ribs. As you lace your belly, pull your ribs strongly in, decreasing the girth of your lower rib cage. Relax your shoulders, which will tend to tense. **(6-1c)**

❻ On the next exhale, relax, allowing your abdominal wall and pelvic floor to expand naturally.

❼ Perform five repetitions.

GOALS

- Teaches the body to contract the deepest abdominal muscle—the transversus abdominus.

- Closes the midline of the body.

- Begins to flatten the abdominal wall.

TRAINING TIPS

If you have trouble breathing, you are contracting your diaphragm and/or tensing your rib cage. Try to relax your upper body. As you gain experience, your body will learn to discriminate between the diaphragm, the chest muscles, and the transversus, and you will be able to isolate one without the others automatically contracting.

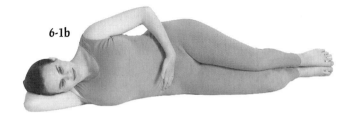

6-1a

6-1b

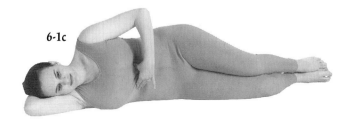

6-1c

Lower Back Release (6-2)

❶ Start in the hollow tuck position. Put one hand under each knee. Tighten your abdominal wall and pull your belly button toward your spine. Contract your pelvic floor muscles.

❷ Using your arms, slowly pull your thighs closer to your chest. Allow your tailbone to curl up toward the ceiling. Deepen the contraction of your abdominal wall, pulling your belly button as close to your spine as possible. Keep your upper spine long and pressed into the floor, your shoulder tips pressed lightly toward the floor, the back of your head lengthened away from your torso. Breathe deeply, allowing your lower back to expand farther on each exhale. **(6-2)**

Goals

➨ Stretches the long muscles of the back (erector spinae).

➨ Strengthens, closes, and flattens the abdominal wall.

➨ Deepens hip flexion.

Training Tips

➨ Always hold under the knees. Holding the tops of the knees and/or the shins overly compresses the cartilage of the knee joints and stresses already lax ligaments.

➨ Try to bring your thighs to your chest rather than bringing your chest to your thighs.

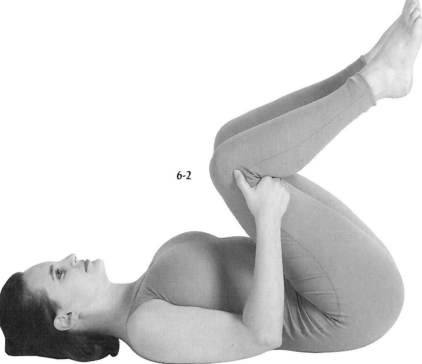

6-2

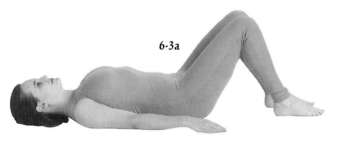

6-3a

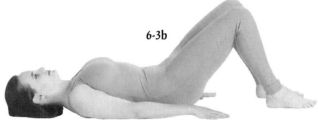

6-3b

Hollow Pelvic Tilt (6-3)

❶ Start in the neutral supine position. Tighten your abdominal wall and pelvic floor muscles. Try to isolate just muscle; don't move bones yet. **(6-3a)**

❷ Anchor your lumbar spine to the floor by simultaneously curling your tailbone toward the ceiling and pulling your belly button as close to your spine as possible. This will hollow your abdominal wall and flatten your lower back. Keep your rib cage relaxed and breathe normally. Relax your shoulders and neck as you exhale. Focus the work between your pubic bone and waist. Keep your gluteals (butt) relaxed.

❸ Exhale; deepen your abdominal contraction. Visualize doing this exercise on sand; don't let your feet indent the sand. Instead, indent the sand with your lower back. Deepen the contraction of your pelvic floor. **(6-3b)**

❹ Exhale; release all muscular effort, allowing your pelvis to gently roll into the neutral position. Your bikini triangle should be flat.

❺ Perform five repetitions.

GOALS

➤ Trains the transversus to synergistically contract with the obliques, the first step in creating dynamic stability.

➤ Shortens the distance between the pubic bone and the waist.

➤ Lengthens the lower back muscles.

➤ Corrects the anterior tilt of the pelvis.

TRAINING TIPS

➤ Pelvic tilts are commonly done by squeezing the gluteals first. However, the gluteals are a power muscle group and should not be used to align or stabilize the inclination of the pelvis. You want to train the abdominals for that job.

➤ You may tend to tighten your diaphragm and/or shoulders. Take a second to let go of unnecessary tension. Breathe deeply.

Single Leg Stretch (6-4)

❶ Start in the neutral supine position. Anchor your spine with a hollow pelvic tilt. Without wobbling, bring your right knee and then your left knee to your chest. Put your left hand under your left knee to help support your leg. Press your shoulder tips down toward the floor. Flex both feet. Put your right heel on the floor. **(6-4a)**

❷ Slide your right heel along the floor, straight out and away from your body. Keep your pelvis stable; don't wobble or give up any of the hollow pelvic tilt. Your leg may not straighten all the way. Keep your rib cage and shoulders relaxed, the back of your neck long. **(6-4b)**

❸ Slowly drag your right heel back in and then bring your right leg into your chest without wobbling your pelvis. Put both hands under your right knee. Repeat on the other side.

❹ Perform twice on each side.

GOALS

➥ Strengthens and flattens the abdominals.

➥ Lengthens the hip flexors (ilio-psoas).

TRAINING TIPS

As your leg slides away from your body, your pubic bone will tend to follow and you will lose the hollow pelvic tilt. Focus on your abdominals and the press of your lower back into the floor. You want to find as much oppositional force as possible without the weight and strength of your leg overpowering your abdominal wall.

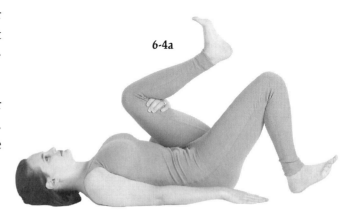

6-4a

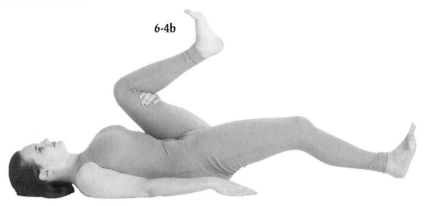

6-4b

Heel Slides (6-5)

❶ Start in the hollow pelvic tilt position. Flex your right foot. **(6-5a)**

❷ Push your right heel along the floor, straight out from your body. Make sure your hips stay stable and your lower back stays firmly pressed into the floor. Your right leg may not straighten all the way. Keep your left leg relaxed. **(6-5b)**

❸ Slowly drag your right heel back in. Again, you want to focus on pelvic stability. Place your foot back on the floor.

❹ Repeat on the left side.

❺ Perform eight repetitions.

GOALS

➥ Flattens the abdominal wall.

➥ Develops dynamic stability.

Focus on the position of your pelvis. It is tempting to shift the pelvis to the side or to press into the bent leg as you initiate the slide and/or the drag-in. Teach yourself to perform a heel slide without shifting your center of gravity. If you feel too much friction, try wearing socks to help facilitate the slide.

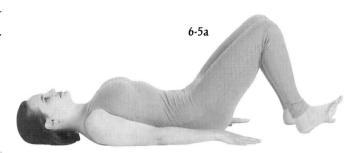

6-5a

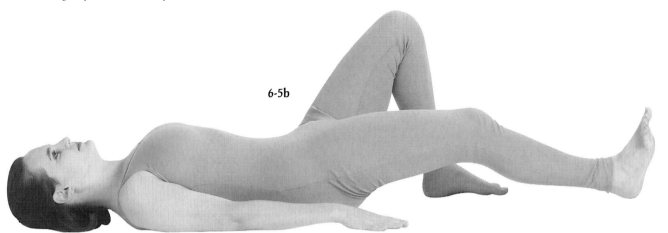

6-5b

Small Toe Taps (6-6)

❶ Start in the hollow pelvic tilt position. Bring one knee and then the other up to the chest without wobbling your pelvis. Allow your lower legs and feet to relax. Reassert the hollow pelvic tilt so that your abdominals are as flat and pulled in as possible. Keep your shoulders relaxed and the back of your neck long. This is the hollow tuck position. See page 26 for greater detail. (**6-6a**)

❷ Without changing the position of your spine, allow one knee to slowly extend away from your chest so that your toe lowers toward the floor. Keep your leg relaxed. If you pass the limit of your functional stability, your pubic bone will begin to follow your thigh. Don't let this occur. Move your knee away from your body only as far as you can maintain complete stability. (**6-6b**)

❸ Slowly pull your knee back up to your chest, still without moving your pelvis.

❹ Repeat eight times on one leg and then eight times on the other leg. Repeat entire sequence twice.

GOALS

➤ Trains the deep abdominal layers to function as stabilizers and work synergistically with the hip flexors.

➤ Strengthens the hip flexors.

TRAINING TIPS

➤ Imagine that you are a marionette and that all of your strings are being pulled taut, especially your belly and pelvis strings. The only string that pulls and releases is the knee string on the working leg.

➤ It is critical to do this exercise without moving the pelvis or allowing the abdominals to bulge. Most postpartum women find that their initial range of functional control is quite small. Don't worry. As you gain strength and co-ordination, you can slowly increase your range of motion.

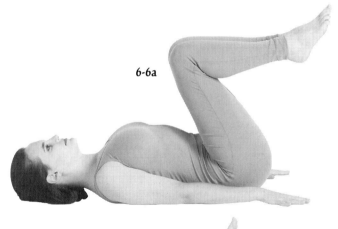

6-6a

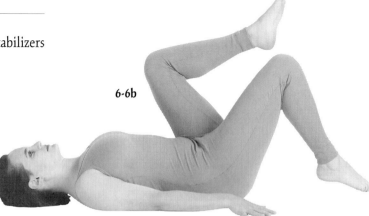

6-6b

Gentle Shoulder Stretch (6-7)

❶ Start in the neutral supine position. Raise both arms above your chest and clasp your hands around your elbows. (Right hand holds left elbow, left hand holds right elbow.) **(6-7a)**

❷ Press both shoulder blades down your back so that your shoulder tips move away from your ears and closer to the floor. Tighten your abdominal wall.

❸ Pull your right elbow left, across the midline of your body, opening the back of your right shoulder girdle. Take care that your shoulder tips do not creep up toward your ears. **(6-7b)**

❹ Breathe into the stretch for thirty seconds.

❺ Repeat on the other side.

GOALS

➥ Stretches overly tight muscles of the shoulder.

➥ Helps align the shoulder girdle.

TRAINING TIPS

Because the muscles that elevate the shoulders are chronically tight after pregnancy, it is easy to let the shoulders hunch up. Keep them pressed down and away from your ears.

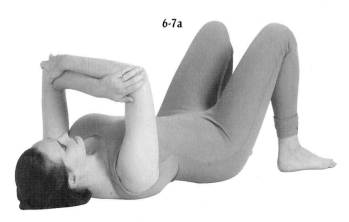

6-7a

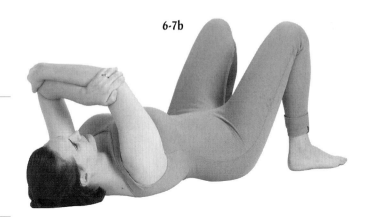

6-7b

Rib Closure (6-8)

❶ Start in the hollow pelvic tilt position. Place your arms at the sides of your body, your palms facing in.

❷ Lift both arms straight off the floor to a high diagonal; hands should stay shoulder width apart. (Your arms will make an arc in space.) Keep your shoulder blades pressed down your back so that they stay neutral. You will be able to see your hands in your peripheral vision.

❸ Exhale, firmly contract your abdominal wall, and narrow the bottom of your rib cage as you stretch your arms higher. (Shoulder blades stay down.) Visualize a wide belt cinching your lower ribs and the fibers of your abdominal wall sliding together. **(6-8)**

❹ Flip your palms to face out and circle your arms to the side and down to return to the starting position.

❺ Repeat five times.

GOALS

→ Flattens the abdominal wall and narrows the waist.

→ Closes the midline and the lower ribs.

→ Stabilizes the upper spine.

→ Teaches good upper body mechanics.

TRAINING TIPS

→ This exercise prepares the body for lifting, carrying, and many of the advanced exercises in this book. Often, as we lift our arms, our shoulder blades hyperextend upward and/or our ribs hyperextend out and pull away from the floor. Test your body as you do this exercise. Typically, your ribs and/or shoulders will lose their placement as your hands approach or pass 90 degrees. Move your arms slowly so that you can feel the stability in your shoulder girdle and rib cage.

→ During the last half of pregnancy, the lower ribs flare out to create more room for the lungs and internal organs. Closing the ribs is an important component of remodeling the waistline.

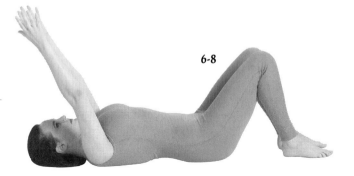

6-8

Exercise After Pregnancy: How to Look and Feel Your Best

Gentle Spiral Stretch (6-9)

❶ Start in the neutral supine position, your arms out to the side. Roll your upper arm bones back so that your inner arms face the ceiling (exterior rotation). Tighten your abdominal wall. Your pelvis remains neutral. **(6-9a)**

❷ Move your left thigh toward your right so that your knees touch (interior rotation). Keep both feet on the floor. Continue pressing your left thigh across as your pelvis begins to twist to the right. Make sure that your back does not arch and your rib cage does not splay upward.

❸ Deepen the spiral by gently pressing your knees toward the floor. Keep your left arm in contact with the floor. Pull your abdominal wall back toward your spine and then stretch your spine by pushing your top (left) hip down and away from your ribs. Both feet stay on the floor. You will feel this stretch where you are tight—in your hips, lower back, or the front of your chest. **(6-9b)**

❹ Breathe into the stretch for thirty seconds. Take care that the stretch is not too intense.

❺ Return your pelvis and knees to the starting position. Exhale, release all muscular effort, and relax for a few moments in the neutral position.

❻ Repeat on the other side.

GOALS

➤ Stretches overly tight muscles.

➤ Mobilizes the spinal column.

➤ Aligns the pelvis and spine.

TRAINING TIPS

➤ Move slowly. Stop and breathe into extra-tight areas. Back off a little if the stretch becomes too intense. You want to be able to maintain the position for a full thirty seconds.

➤ If you are tight in the front of your chest, your upper arm will roll inward. Keep your inner arms facing the ceiling.

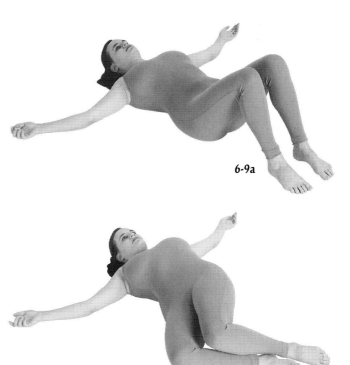

6-9a

6-9b

Hamstring Stretch (6-10)

❶ Start in the neutral supine position. Tighten your abdominal wall. Straighten your right leg to a 45-degree angle with the floor. Strongly flex your right foot and then lift your right leg higher until you begin to feel a stretch on the back of your leg. Keep your knee straight, thigh muscles tight, and pelvis neutral. Maintain the stretch for ten slow counts. (**6-10**)

❷ Repeat on the left side.

❸ Repeat each side three times, alternating sides.

GOALS

➤ Lengthens the hamstrings.

➤ Increases hip flexion.

➤ Strengthens the thighs.

➤ Centers and stabilizes the pelvis.

TRAINING TIPS

Most of us try to stretch the hamstrings in positions that also curve the lower spine. To gain hip flexion and true hamstring length, it is important to stabilize the pelvis in the neutral position. Your bikini triangle will remain parallel to the floor and your lumbar curve will remain intact. Use your abdominals to maintain pelvis placement.

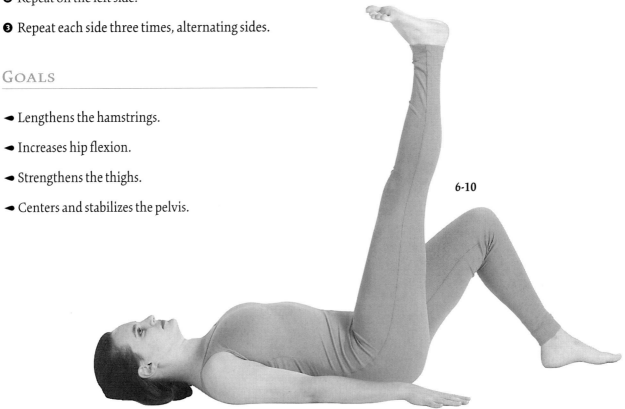

6-10

Half Cat (6-11)

❶ Start in the quadruped position. Your spine is neutral, your thighs and arms perpendicular to the floor. Your knees are four to six inches apart, shins parallel, and feet relaxed. Firmly push away from the floor with your arms and slide your shoulder blades down your back. Lengthen the back of your neck, rotating your chin toward your chest. **(6-11a)**

❷ Lift your belly strongly to your spine. Curl your tailbone under as you deepen the lift of your belly (a hollow pelvic tilt). Take care to isolate only your lower spine. Your upper spine (thorax, neck, and head) remains neutral. Breathe normally. **(6-11b)**

❸ Holding your abdominal wall as tight and close to your spine as possible, slowly unfurl your pelvis into the neutral position. Be careful not to sag through your arms, shoulders, or waist.

❹ Repeat five times.

GOALS

➽ Flattens the abdominal wall.

➽ Lengthens the lower back.

➽ Stabilizes the upper spine and shoulder girdle.

TRAINING TIPS

➽ It can be difficult to isolate the lower spine in this position. You may find yourself pushing back through your upper spine. Because pregnancy leaves you overly kyphotic, this movement is not appropriate right now.

➽ This exercise is commonly taught by moving the spine into a complete hyperextension, which shortens the lower back and stretches the abdominal wall. Again, this movement is not desirable in the postpartum period. Hence, we perform a Half Cat rather than a Full Cat. Concentrate on maintaining a neutral upper spine and shoulders.

➽ If you experience any wrist pain, use your fists rather than your palms to support your upper body in the quadruped position. You can also do this exercise standing up.

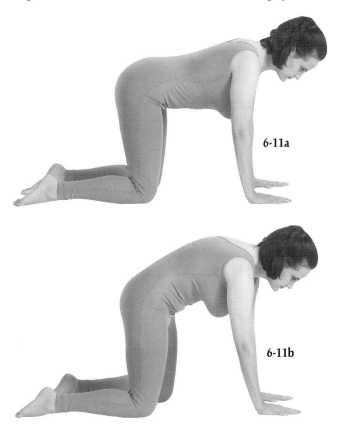

6-11a

6-11b

Hunting Dog (6-12)

❶ Start in the quadruped position. Your spine is neutral, arms and thighs perpendicular to the floor, shoulders pressed firmly down your back, neck elongated. Tighten your abdominal wall and pull your belly away from the floor as much as you can without disrupting the neutral spine. **(6-12a)**

❷ Slide your right foot out along the floor without wobbling or changing the position of your spine. Continue extending your leg and lift your foot off the floor, straightening your leg behind you. **(6-12b)**

❸ Slide your left hand forward along the floor and extend your arm off the floor. Your hand and foot will be slightly lower than the rest of your body. Make sure your hips stay parallel to the floor and your waist does not sag. Balance for eight slow counts. **(6-12c)**

❹ Smoothly bring your hand and foot back into the quadruped position.

❺ Repeat on the other side.

❻ Repeat both sides twice.

GOALS

➡ Trains the abdominals and back muscles to function synergistically to support a neutral spine.

➡ Develops kinesthetic awareness.

TRAINING TIPS

➡ Keep your pelvis absolutely still. Your leg stays in parallel position (knee faces the floor) and will not lift very high. If you need to make an adjustment as you return to the quadruped position, you did not maintain a neutral spine.

➡ Keep your shoulder blades firmly pressed down your back so they do not hyperextend as you reach out.

➡ Move slowly and smoothly so you can tune in to what your body is doing.

➡ If you experience wrist pain, use fists to support your upper body. If the fist variation is uncomfortable, do not perform this exercise.

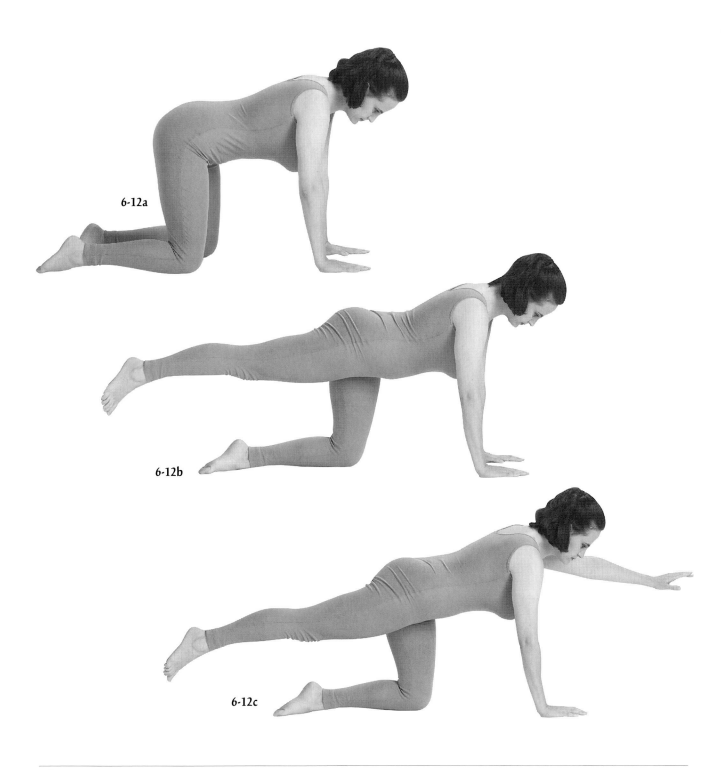

6-12a

6-12b

6-12c

Neck Stretch (6-13)

❶ Sit tall with your legs in a relaxed diamond position or a relaxed "tailor" position (shins crossed). Your pelvis should be in the neutral position, your bikini triangle vertical, so that you're right on top of your sits bone (ischium). Pull your abdominals firmly in and elongate your spine. Lengthen the back of your head up and back so that your ears align over your shoulders. Rotate your chin toward your chest. **(6-13a)**

❷ Pull your left shoulder blade an inch or so down your back without moving your spine. **(6-13b)**

❸ Tilt your head to the right. Breathe into the stretch for eight slow counts. Be sure to keep your spine stable. Your rib cage does not move. **(6-13c)**

❹ Deepen the stretch by pulling your left shoulder farther down your back. Release the muscular effort and allow your head to float back into the neutral position.

❺ Repeat on the other side.

❻ Repeat each side twice.

GOALS

→ Aligns the upper spine, shoulder girdle, and head.

→ Releases tight shoulder and neck muscles.

→ Teaches the abdominal and lower back muscles to stabilize the neutral position.

TRAINING TIPS

→ The muscle that pulls the shoulder girdle down the back (serratus anterior) can be difficult to find at first. Your shoulder tip will move down only an inch or so. Look in a mirror to see your shoulder tip move down while your ribs remain still.

→ Strength in the serratus anterior is an important component of functional balance in the shoulder girdle and of ergonomic lifting and carrying.

Exercise After Pregnancy: How to Look and Feel Your Best

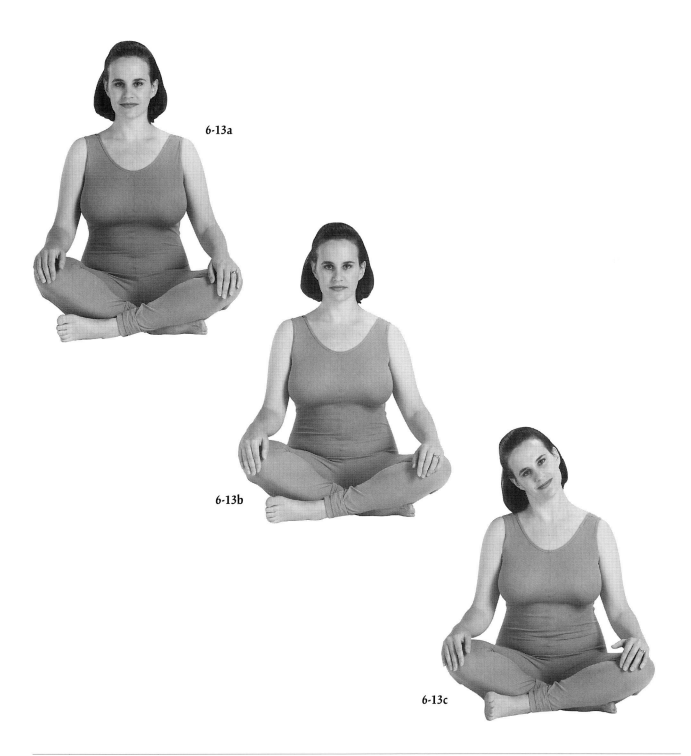

6-13a

6-13b

6-13c

Chapter Seven

Step Two:
Knitting Back Together

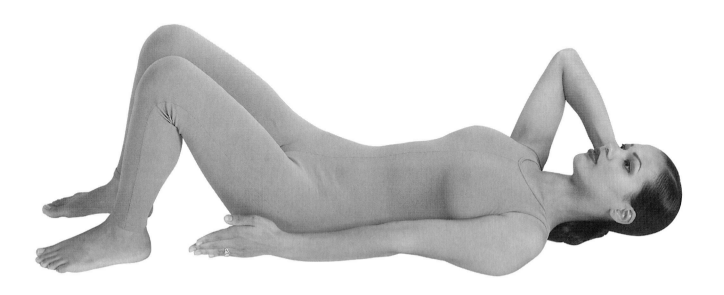

THE FOLLOWING EXERCISES build on the techniques and principles introduced in Chapter Six. Even if you are no longer postpartum, do not start your exercise program here. Spend several weeks practicing the exercises in Chapter Six so that your body is prepared for the work in this section.

As you learn the following exercises, pay attention to your abdominal wall and the position of your pelvis. After pregnancy, the weight and strength of the limbs often overpower the functional capacity of the abdominal wall, causing it to balloon outward and/or the pelvis to lose stability. Work within the range of motion that is appropriate for your body. Gradually increase your range of motion as your strength increases. Always focus on quality over quantity. Plan on staying at this level for at least three months or until the exercises no longer challenge your body.

Spiral Stretch (7-1)

❶ Start in the neutral supine position, your arms out to the side. Roll your upper arms back so that your inner arms face the ceiling (exterior rotation). Tighten your abdominal wall. **(7-1a)**

❷ Move your left thigh toward your right so that your knees touch (interior rotation). Keep both feet on the floor. Continue pressing your left thigh across as your pelvis begins to twist right. Make sure your upper back does not arch and your ribs do not splay upward.

❸ Deepen the spiral by dragging your left leg over your right until your left knee passes your right knee. Keep your left foot on the floor as you straighten your left knee. Keep your left arm in contact with the floor. You will feel this

stretch where you are tight—in the hips, lower back, and chest. Take care that the stretch is not too intense. **(7-1b)**

❹ Breathe into the stretch for thirty seconds.

❺ Bend your left leg and return your pelvis and legs to the starting position. Release all muscular effort and relax for a few moments in the neutral position.

❻ Repeat on the other side.

GOALS

➥ Elongates and mobilizes the spine.

➥ Releases overly tight muscle groups.

➥ Improves alignment.

TRAINING TIPS

➥ Move slowly. Try to articulate one vertebra at a time. Breathe into any tight areas.

➥ If you are tight in the chest, your upper arm will roll inward. Keep your inner arms facing the ceiling. Keep your neck long and your head neutral.

➥ If you are not feeling enough stretch in your chest, raise your arms slightly to above shoulder height.

➥ If you are tight in the gluteals, your top foot will tend to pull off the floor. Bend your knee and allow your top thigh to rest on your bottom thigh.

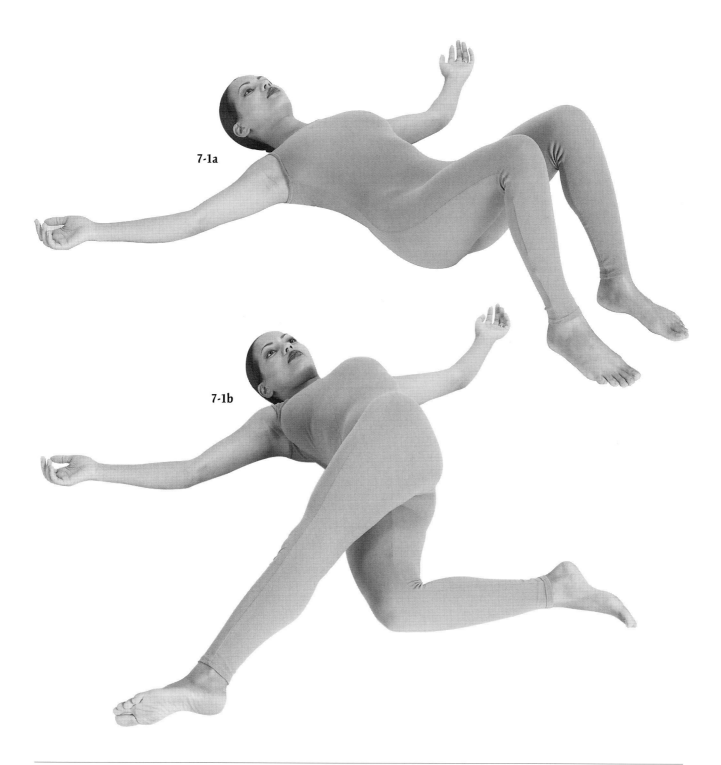

7-1a

7-1b

Shoulder Stretch (7-2)

❶ Start in the neutral supine position; rest your hands on your lower rib cage.

❷ Inhale deeply. On the exhale, float your left arm straight up to the ceiling, keeping your shoulder girdle neutral. **(7-2a)**

❸ Inhale deeply. On the exhale, move your left shoulder blade out and away from your spine and reach your left arm closer to the ceiling, stretching your upper back muscles. Your left shoulder tip should move down and away from your left ear, not hunch up.

❹ Inhale deeply, maintaining the stretch. Exhale, push your left shoulder blade farther out, and reach your left arm farther toward the ceiling. **(7-2b)**

❺ Deepen the breathing/stretch sequence a third time.

❻ Inhale deeply. On the exhale, release all muscular effort, allowing your left shoulder to drop onto the floor; your left hand comes to rest on your lower ribs.

❼ Repeat on the right side.

❽ Repeat entire sequence, left and right sides, once.

GOALS

● Stretches the upper back muscles.

● Aligns the shoulder girdle.

● Aligns the upper spine and head.

TRAINING TIPS

● Your shoulder tip will tend to creep toward your ear as you slide your shoulder blade away from your spine. Focus on moving your shoulder tip down and away from your ear.

● Keep your spine and rib cage absolutely stable, the back of your neck long.

● This is a great stretch for relieving shoulder spasms.

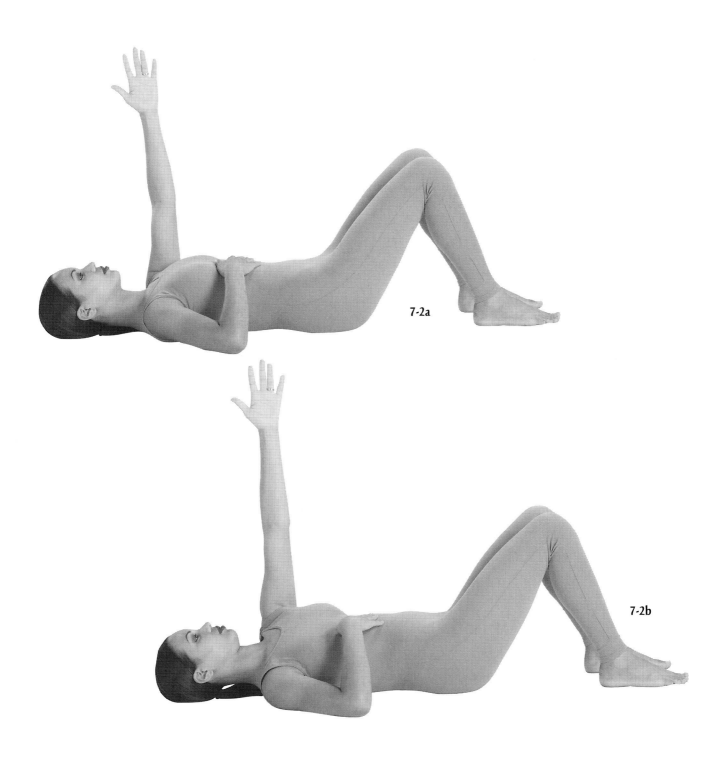

7-2a

7-2b

Flat Bridges (7-3)

❶ Start in the neutral supine position. Tighten your lower abdominal wall and move into a hollow pelvic tilt. **(7-3a)**

❷ Continue deepening the work of your abdominals as your pelvis lifts off the floor. Slowly roll your vertebrae, one at a time, off the floor until your spine (except for your neck and head) is on a long diagonal—a flat bridge position. Keep your abdominal wall pulled in as tightly as possible and your rib cage and shoulders relaxed. Take care that your thighs remain parallel and your knees stay directly over your feet. **(7-3b)**

❸ Maintain the flat bridge through two long breath cycles, all the while elongating your spine and pulling your weight out of your lower back. You may feel your gluteals and hamstrings work intensely.

❹ Slowly lower your spine one vertebra at a time, all the while pulling your tailbone toward the ceiling. Deepen your abdominal hollowing on the way down. **(7-3c)**

❺ When your lower spine is back on the floor, exhale deeply and release all muscular effort, and allow your pelvis to roll into the neutral position.

❻ Repeat five times.

Goals

➨ Strengthens the lower abdominals.

➨ Develops spine articulation.

➨ Strengthens the gluteals and the hamstrings.

Training Tips

➨ Keep your lower ribs pulled in; they will tend to flare out at the top of the bridge.

➨ As you articulate your spine, particularly on the way down, your shoulders will tend to hunch up. Press your shoulder tips to the floor so that they stay neutral.

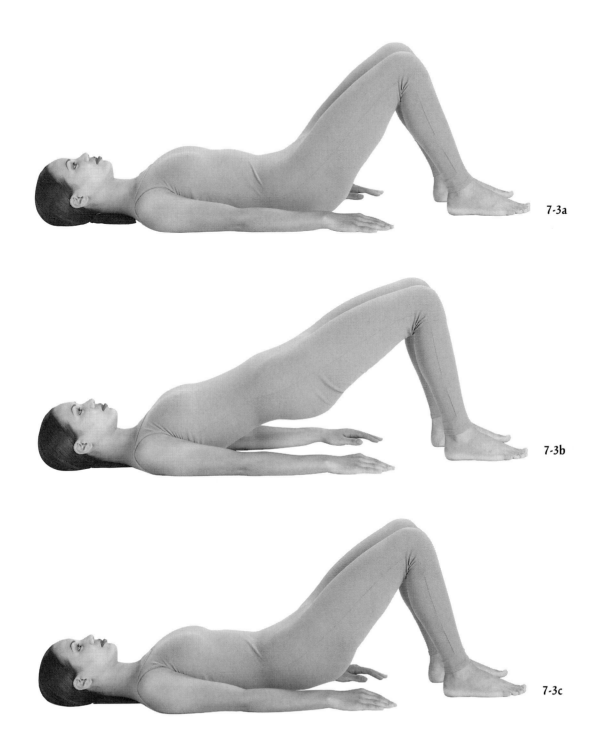

7-3a

7-3b

7-3c

Alternating Toe Taps (7-4)

❶ Start in the hollow pelvic tilt position. Bring one knee and then the other to your chest without wobbling your pelvis. Relax your lower legs and feet. Reassert the hollow pelvic tilt so that your abdominals are as tight as possible. Keep your shoulders relaxed and the back of your neck long. (This is the hollow tuck position.) **(7-4a)**

❷ Without changing the position of your spine, slowly extend your right knee away from your chest until your toe lightly touches the floor. **(7-4b)**

❸ Slowly pull your right knee back up to your chest as your left knee begins to extend and tap on the other side. Your legs will work in opposition as if on a pulley system. **(7-4c)**

❹ Perform a total of sixteen taps. Rest briefly in the neutral position.

❺ Repeat the entire sequence once.

GOALS

→ Strengthens the hip flexors.

→ Trains the obliques and tranversus to function as stabilizers.

→ Teaches the legs and spine to function independently of each other.

TRAINING TIPS

→ Many postpartum women will not be able to touch their toe to the floor while maintaining a hollow pelvic tilt and a stable pelvis. Test yourself so that you can determine your appropriate range of motion. As you develop strength and coordination, gradually increase your range of motion until your toes can touch the floor.

→ Imagine that you are a marionette and that all of your strings are being pulled taut, especially the belly and pubic bone strings. As you tap, the only strings that release are the knee strings.

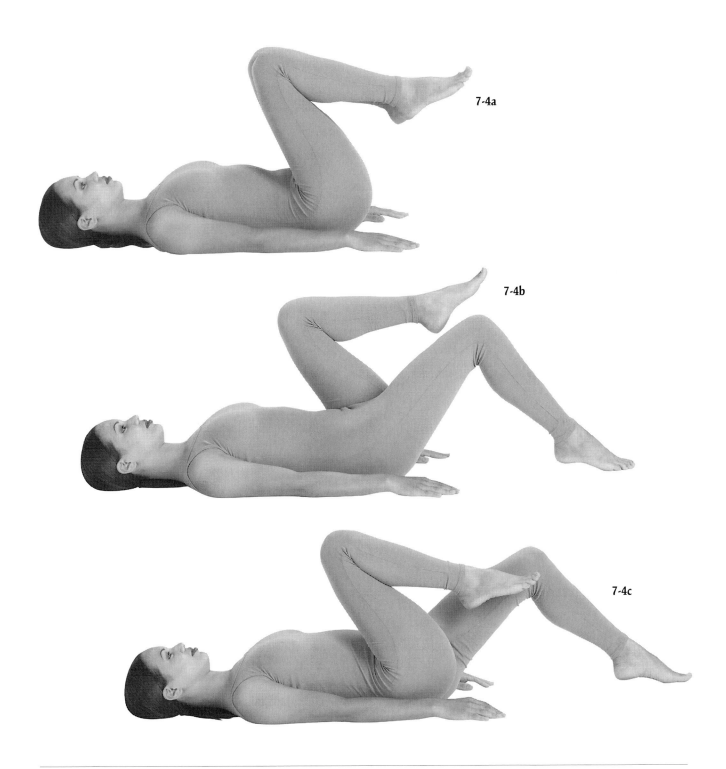

7-4a

7-4b

7-4c

Small Leg Arcs (7-5)

❶ Start in the hollow pelvic tilt position. Bring one knee and then the other into your chest without wobbling your pelvis (the hollow tuck position). Flex both feet. Straighten your right leg so that it is perpendicular to the floor. **(7-5a)**

❷ Slowly, in two counts, lower your right leg toward the floor as you pull your left knee closer to your chest. Go only as far as you can control. Take care that your pubic bone does not follow the right leg and that your abdominal wall stays flat. **(7-5b)**

❸ Bend your right knee and pull your right thigh back to your chest. Reassert the abdominal hollowing.

❹ Extend your left leg up, and repeat on the other side.

❺ Perform eight alternating leg arcs on each side.

GOALS

→ Strengthens the hip flexors.

→ Strengthens and flattens the abdominal wall.

→ Develops synergistic functioning of the legs and abdominals.

TRAINING TIPS

→ Try to keep your gesture leg straight.

→ This is a two-leg exercise. Work both legs equally in opposition.

→ As stability exercises begin to get challenging, the shoulders and neck tend to tighten. Keep your shoulders relaxed and the back of your neck long.

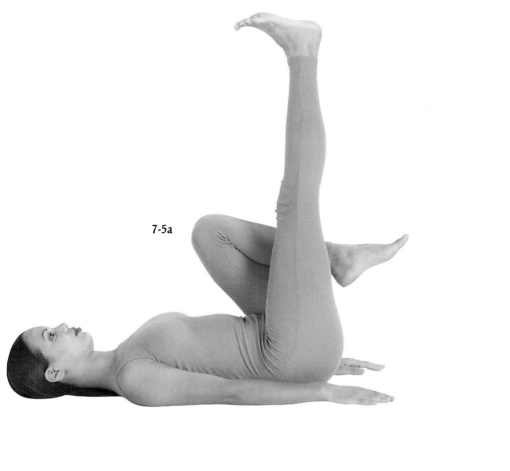

7-5a

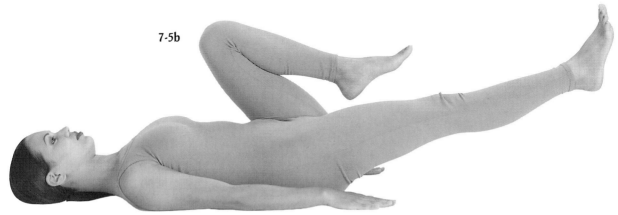

7-5b

Small Reverse Curls (7-6)

❶ Start in the hollow tuck position. Lift both legs to form a 90-degree angle, thighs vertical and shins parallel to the floor. **(7-6a)**

❷ Roll your lower spine off the floor by contracting your lower abdominals. You don't have to go very high. Hold the top of the curl for a moment. **(7-6b)**

❸ Roll down slowly. Tilt your legs slightly to your left side, keeping both sides of your pelvis in contact with the floor. **(7-6c)**

❹ Roll your lower spine off the floor with your legs to the left side. Hold the top of the curl for a moment. **(7-6d)**

❺ Roll down slowly. Repeat with legs centered and to the right side.

❻ Perform eight sets (center, left, center, right).

Strengthens the lower abdominals.

TRAINING TIPS

You may not be able to lift your pelvis off the floor at first. Start with a small range of motion you can control. It's okay if your knees straighten slightly, but be careful not to use the momentum of the legs to get your pelvis off the floor.

7-6a

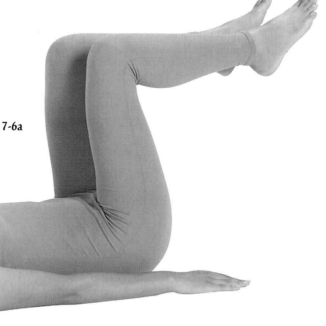

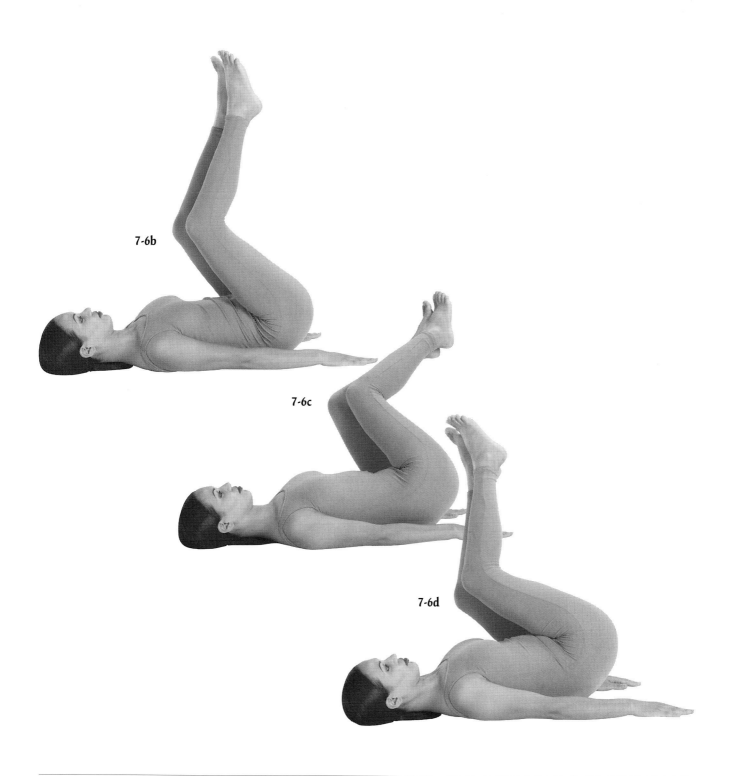

7-6b

7-6c

7-6d

For the next two exercises, select either Classic Crunches and Oblique Pulses, or Crunches with Abdominal Splinting and Oblique Pulses with Abdominal Splinting.

Classic Crunches (7-7)

❶ Start in the hollow pelvic tilt position. Press your shoulder blades down your back. Put your hands, fingers splayed, behind your head and neck. Rotate your head so that the back of your neck lengthens and your chin moves toward your chest. Your elbows are on a 45-degree diagonal within your peripheral vision; shoulders are neutral. **(7-7a)**

❷ Roll your head and shoulders off the floor by moving your rib cage toward the pelvis. Keep your chin the same distance from your chest throughout the crunch. Try not to flex your neck or pull with your elbows. All movement should come from your lower ribs.

❸ At the top of the crunch, pull your belly in deeper toward your spine. **(7-7b)**

❹ Roll down slowly, hollowing out your abdominals more. Elongate the back of your neck as you roll down.

❺ Perform sixteen repetitions.

GOALS

➥ Strengthens the abdominal wall, especially the upper half.

➥ Flattens and closes the abdominal wall.

➥ Trains the transversus to function synergistically with the rectus and obliques.

TRAINING TIPS

➥ If you have abdominal separation, perform Crunches with Abdominal Splinting instead (see next exercise).

➥ If your abdominal wall bulges, your transversus is not strong enough yet. Use a smaller range of motion and focus on hollowing your belly on the way up and down.

➥ If you experience neck pain, see the abdominal wall training techniques in Chapter Five.

Exercise After Pregnancy: How to Look and Feel Your Best

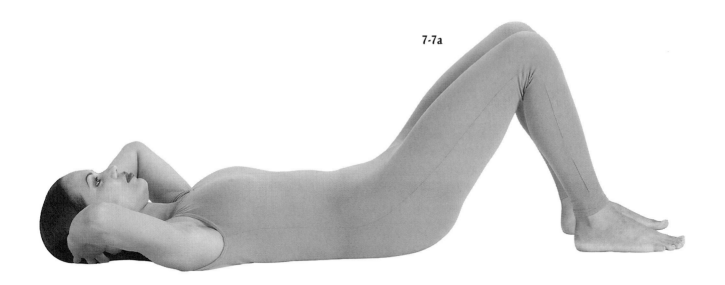

7-7a

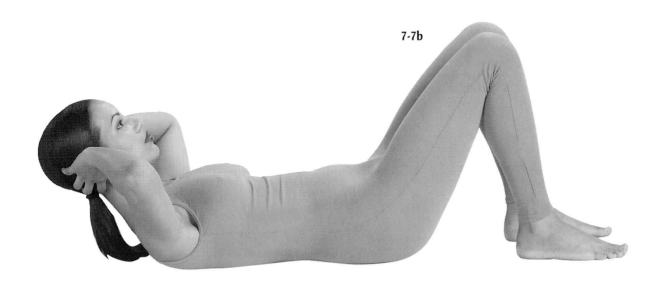

7-7b

Crunches
with Abdominal Splinting (7-8)

❶ Prepare the body in the same way as for Classic Crunches, but use your fingers to push the recti muscles together toward your midline. **(7-8a)**

❷ Roll your head and shoulders off the floor by moving your rib cage toward your pelvis, using the pressure of your fingers to manually close the abdominal separation. At the top of the crunch, pull your belly in deeper toward your spine. **(7-8b)**

❸ Roll down slowly, hollowing out your abdominals more.

❹ Perform eight repetitions. Rest your head on the floor (keeping the back of your neck long) for a few moments to relieve your neck if necessary. Do one more set of eight crunches.

GOALS

➥ Closes abdominal separation.

➥ Strengthens and flattens the abdominal wall.

TRAINING TIPS

Because your hands do not support your head, it is easy to overwork your neck muscles. Focus on maintaining the relationship of your head and neck and motivate the movement from your rib cage. Rest if your neck begins to ache.

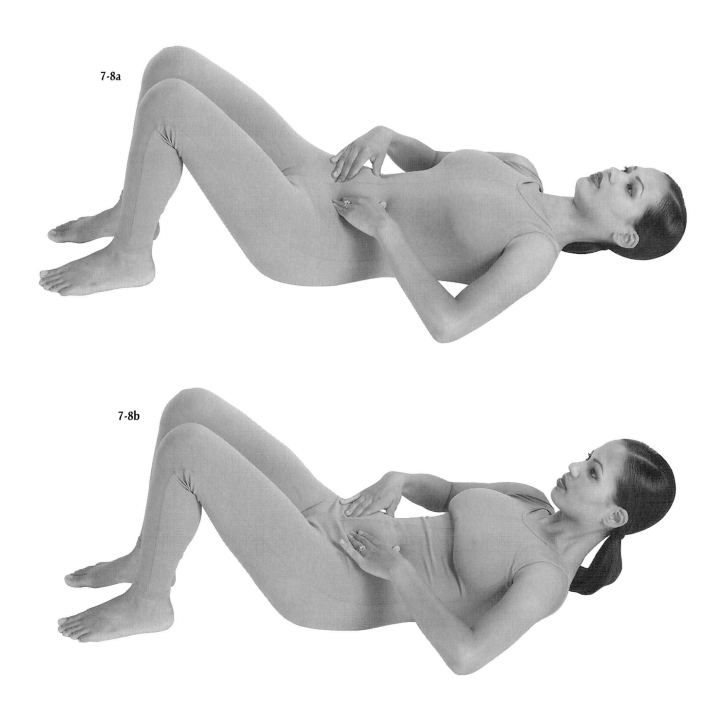

7-8a

7-8b

Oblique Pulses (7-9)

❶ Prepare the body in the same way as for Classic Crunches. Place your right hand behind your head; reach your left arm along the left side of your body. **(7-9a)**

❷ Pull the left side of your rib cage toward the left side of your pelvis by curling your torso to the left. Your left hand will try to touch your left heel. Both shoulder blades will come slightly off the floor. **(7-9b)**

❸ Pulse your rib cage eight times. Make sure that your pelvis stays completely still.

❹ Return your torso to center and change arms. Repeat on the right side.

❺ Perform four sets, left and right.

● Strengthens the obliques.

● Flattens the abdominal wall.

● If you have abdominal separation, perform Oblique Pulses with Abdominal Splinting instead (see next exercise).

● Take care that your pelvis does not begin to rock in response to the pulse and that your abdominal wall stays flat.

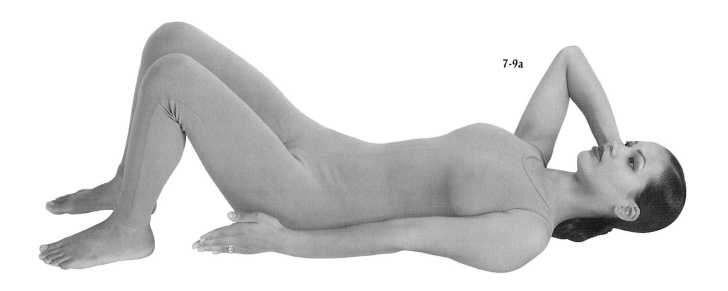

7-9a

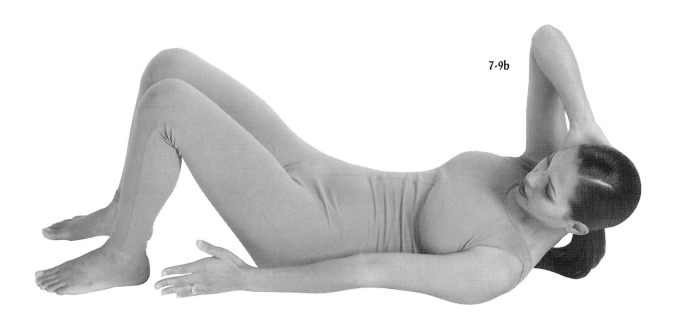

7-9b

Oblique Pulses
with Abdominal Splinting (7-10)

❶ Prepare the body in the same way as for Crunches with Abdominal Splinting. **(7-10a)**

❷ Push your recti muscles in toward your midline with your fingers, as you pull the left side of your rib cage toward the left side of your pelvis, curling your torso to the left. Both shoulder blades will come slightly off the floor. **(7-10b)**

❸ Pulse your rib cage eight times. Make sure your pelvis stays completely still.

❹ Perform eight repetitions on each side twice.

GOALS

➡ Closes the midline.

➡ Strengthens and flattens the abdominal wall.

TRAINING TIPS

➡ *Do not twist the upper body as you pulse.* Oblique crunches are often taught with twists—the upper spine rotates around its central axis. This action can further separate your midline. Move your torso to a *front diagonal curve* and close the side that you are going toward as you crunch. (Upper body twists during abdominal work are an acceptable and challenging variation for the well-conditioned general population.)

➡ Rest your head on the floor if your neck begins to ache. Use the techniques described in Chapter Five to help stabilize your head and neck.

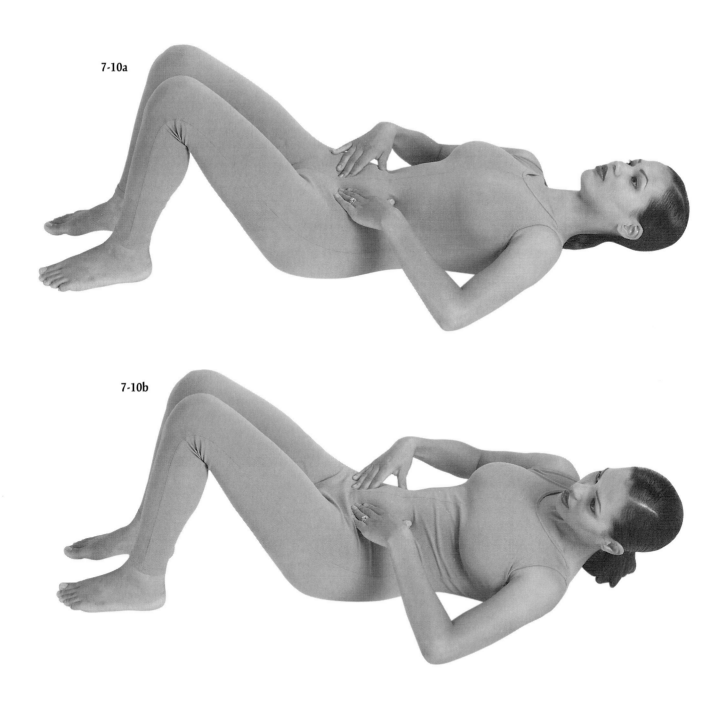

7-10a

7-10b

Half Cobra (7-11)

❶ Lie prone (face down), forehead on the floor, legs close together, feet extended. Place your hands, palms down, next to your shoulders, elbows close to your waist.

❷ Using your abdominal wall (no gluteals), perform a hollow pelvic tilt. Your belly will lift off the floor (or try to) and your pubic bone will contact and anchor to the floor. **(7-11a)**

❸ Lift your head two inches off the floor.

❹ Lift your chest slightly off the floor without using your arms. Slide your shoulder blades down your back and slightly together. Hold the position for four slow counts. **(7-11b)**

❺ Lengthen your spine as you release back down into the starting position.

❻ Perform eight repetitions.

● Strengthens the upper back.

● Improves posture.

● Prepares the body for lifting and carrying.

● For most people, upper back extension is a very small movement. Maintain a strong hollow pelvic tilt so that your lower back (lumbar curve) is supported and does not arch. If you feel any compression in your lower back, pull your abdominals in more firmly and don't go as far off the floor.

● If your breasts are uncomfortable in the prone position, fold a bath towel in quarters lengthwise and then in half crosswise. Lie on the folded towel, with the top of the towel below your breasts, to give yourself a little more room.

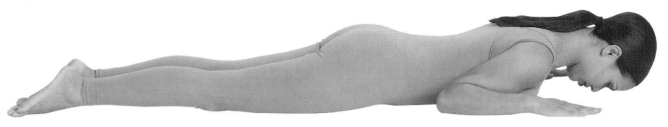

7-11a

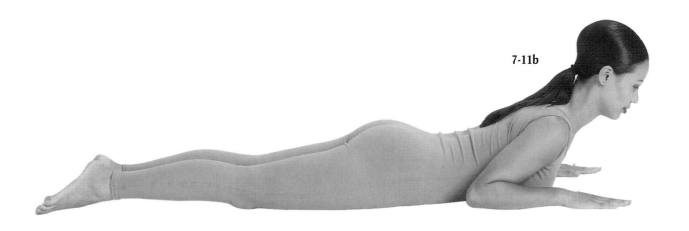

7-11b

Child's Pose (7-12)

❶ From the prone position, fold your body so that your pelvis is close to your heels and your torso is draped onto (or near) your thighs. If you're tight in the hips, place your hands on the floor near your shoulders to help support your body.

❷ Breathe deeply and allow your body (especially your hip sockets) to relax into the stretch for thirty seconds. **(7-12)**

GOALS

- Lengthens the spine.

- Increases hip flexion.

- Releases muscular tension.

TRAINING TIPS

- If getting your hips close to your heels is difficult, start by sitting upright on folded legs and releasing your spine as close to your thighs as you can. You want your hips to be as close to your ankles as possible.

- Press your shoulders firmly down your back so they don't hunch up toward your ears.

- If the deep bend of your knees bothers you, fold a small hand towel in quarters and place it behind your knees to relieve compression. If you continue to feel knee pain, substitute the Half Cat in Chapter Six.

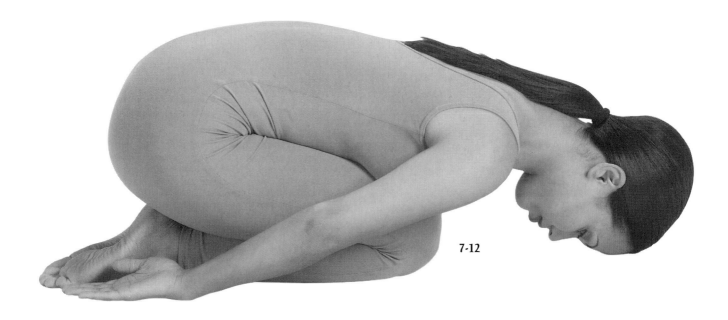

7-12

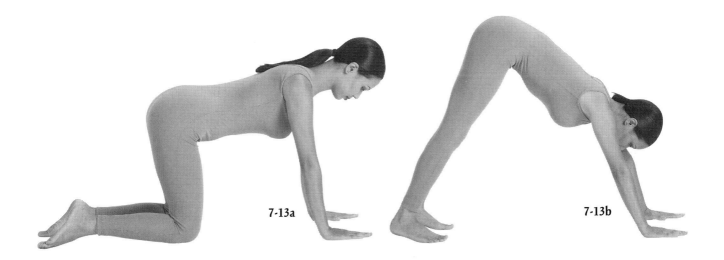

7-13a

7-13b

A-Frame Stretch (7-13)

❶ Start in the quadruped position. **(7-13a)**

❷ Straighten your legs and push your tailbone up toward the ceiling to form an "A." Lift your abdominal wall back toward your spine as much as you can. Push firmly through your shoulders and arms, elongating your torso. Spine stays neutral, lumbar curve intact. Keep your thigh muscles tight, taking care that your knees do not hyperextend. Breathe into the stretch for thirty seconds. **(7-13b)**

❸ Release back into the quadruped position, relax for a few seconds, and repeat the stretch once.

GOALS

➤ Lengthens the hamstrings and calf muscles.

➤ Strengthens the back, shoulders, and arms.

➤ Flattens the abdominal wall.

TRAINING TIPS

➤ Keep your shoulders firmly pressed down your back. Keep the back of your neck long.

➤ Relax the front of your ankles so that your heels lengthen toward the floor.

Sitting Spirals
with Lower Back Stretch (7-14)

❶ Part 1: Sit in either the tailor position (with ankles crossed) or the diamond position (soles of the feet together). Tighten your abdominal wall. Lengthen your spine. Reach your arms out to the sides, slightly in front of your body, and press your shoulder blades down your back. Turn your palms to the ceiling. Bend your elbows, keeping your upper arms parallel to the floor, and touch your fingertips to your shoulders. **(7-14a)**

❷ Slowly rotate your spine right, from the bottom up, around its central axis. Turn your head so that you look over your right shoulder. The distance between your elbows does not change. Upper arms stay parallel to the floor. **(7-14b)**

❸ Pull strongly with your abdominals to recenter your spine.

❹ Repeat the rotation to your left side.

❺ Repeat the rotations to each side three more times.

❻ Part 2: Stay in the last rotation to the right. Place your hands on the floor on either side of your right knee. Bend at your hips so that your torso lengthens and then gently curves over your right knee. You'll get a terrific stretch on the left side of your lower back. **(7-14c)**

❼ Build your spine back up to a neutral sitting position by pulling your abdominals up and into your body. Roll up one vertebra at a time.

❽ Rotate your spine to the left and repeat the lower back stretch to the other side.

GOALS

◗ Strengthens the deep rotators of the spine.

◗ Lengthens the muscles on the lower back and hips.

TRAINING TIPS

◗ If you have pain in the sacroiliac joint (where the back of the pelvis meets the lower spine) do not do Part 2. Keep the spine vertical.

◗ Lengthen the spine throughout the exercise; keep your abdominal wall tight.

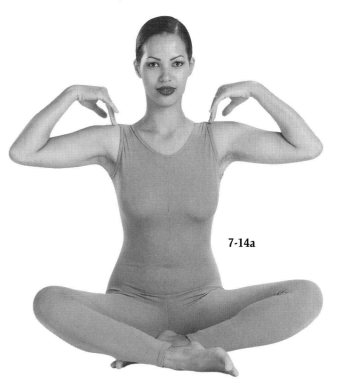

7-14a

Exercise After Pregnancy: How to Look and Feel Your Best

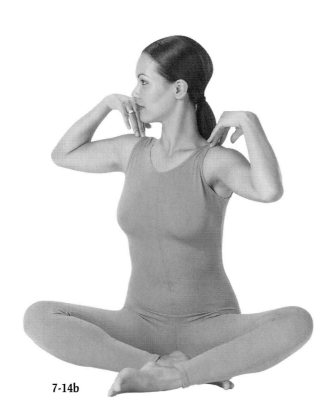

7-14b

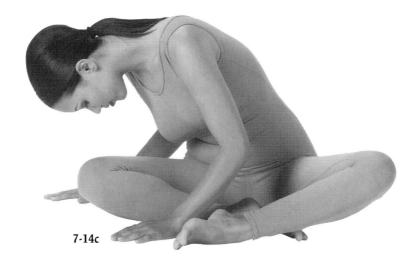

7-14c

Small Squats (7-15)

❶ Stand tall, pelvis neutral, spine long, feet slightly wider than your hips (parallel second). **(7-15a)**

❷ Simultaneously bend your hips, knees, and ankles. Your pubic bone will move backward and your spine will tilt to a high diagonal. Maintain your natural lumbar curve. Don't try to tuck your tailbone under or perform a "flat back." Rest your hands lightly on your thighs.

❸ Continue bending your knees until you feel the work in your quadriceps (thigh muscles). **(7-15b)**

❹ Pulse slightly in the squat, staying as low as you can. Keep your knees over your feet, and the arches of your feet intact. Continue pulsing until you feel your quadriceps fatigue, then rise up to the starting position—pelvis neutral, spine long and supported by the abdominal wall.

❺ Repeat squat/pulse sequence.

GOALS

→ Strengthens the legs, hips, and back.

→ Improves posture.

→ Prepares the body for lifting and carrying.

TRAINING TIPS

→ Start with the number of pulses you can do while maintaining a neutral spine. Slowly add repetitions as you get stronger until you can do thirty-two deep pulses in a row.

→ Take care that your spine does not curve or bob as you tire.

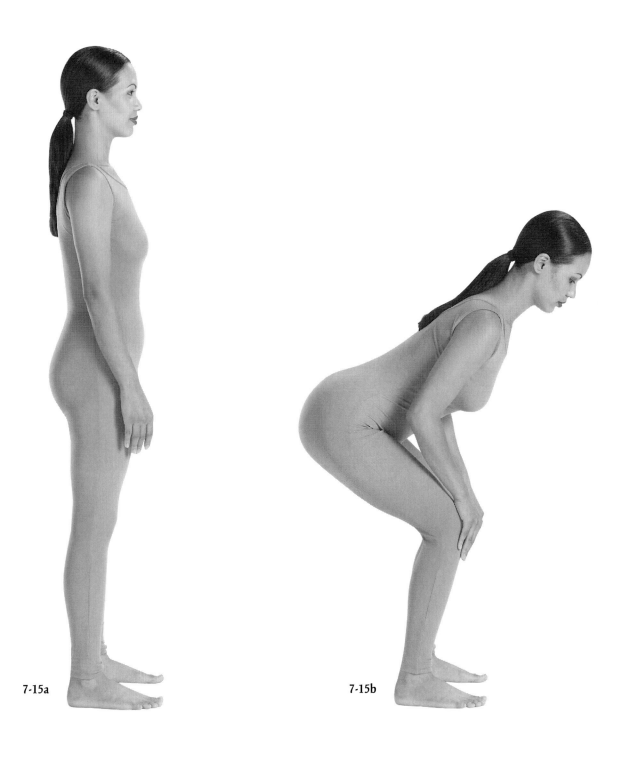

7-15a   7-15b

Chapter Eight

Step Three:
Advanced Core Strength

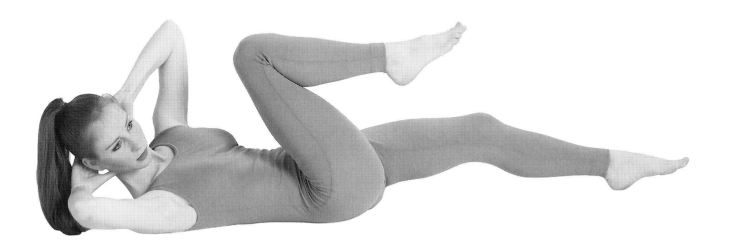

The following exercises assume that you have mastered the basics of dynamic stability—that you can maintain the position of your pelvis during movement and that you have reestablished significant tone in all four layers of the abdominal wall. These exercises are challenging. If at any time you begin to wobble or lose your alignment, or you need to recruit adjoining muscle groups, take a break. To resume, refocus your mental and physical energies and try the exercise with a smaller range of motion. If one or two of the exercises are too challenging, substitute a similar exercise from Chapter Seven.

Elongated Spiral (8-1)

❶ Start in the neutral supine position, arms out to the side. Roll your upper arm bones back so that your inner arms face the ceiling (exterior rotation). Tighten your abdominal wall.

❷ Move your left thigh toward your right so that your knees touch (interior rotation). Keep both feet on the floor. **(8-1a)**

❸ Continue pressing your left thigh across as your pelvis begins to twist to the right. Make sure that your upper back does not arch and that your ribs do not splay upward.

❹ Deepen the spiral by dragging your left leg over your right until your left knee passes your right knee. Keep your left arm in contact with the floor. **(8-1b)**

❺ Elongate the spiral by straightening your left leg, while raising your left hand above your head. Keep your hand and foot on the floor. Press your left hip away from your rib cage. Make sure that your left shoulder does not

hyperextend as you raise your hand. You want to make one line from your left hand to your left foot. Take care that the stretch is not too intense. **(8-1c)**

❻ Breathe into the stretch for thirty seconds.

❼ Bend your left leg, lower your left arm, and return your pelvis to the neutral position, moving your legs into the starting position. Release your spine and relax for a moment in the neutral position with your bikini triangle parallel to the floor.

❽ Repeat on the other side.

GOALS

➡ Elongates and mobilizes the spine.

➡ Releases overly tight muscle groups.

➡ Improves alignment.

TRAINING TIPS

➡ As with the previous spirals, move slowly, articulating one vertebra at a time.

➡ Try to create one long line in space from your toes to your fingertips. Make sure that your spine does not arch and that your shoulders stay neutral. For many, a small raise of the arm can cause an intense stretch in the chest. Respect your body's limits.

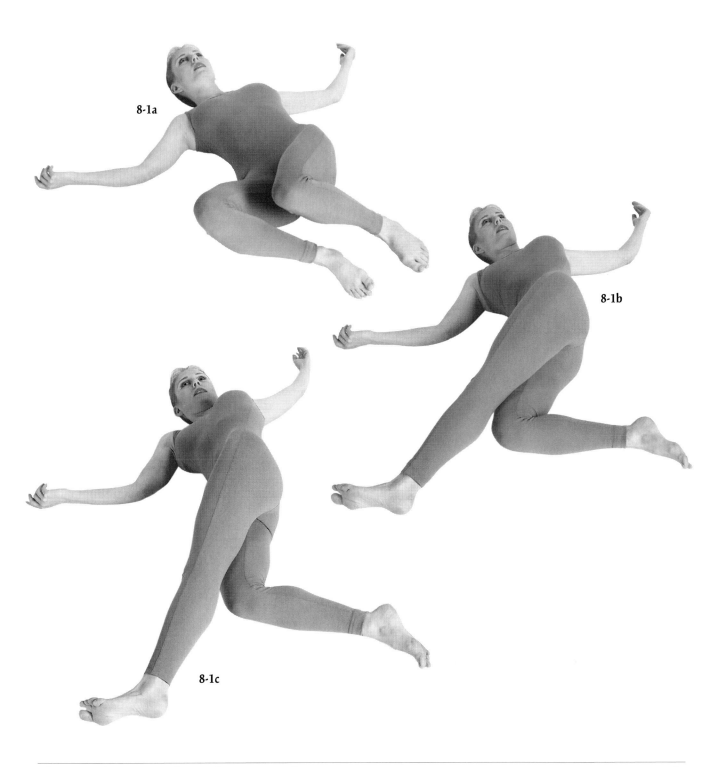

8-1a

8-1b

8-1c

Shoulder Stretch with Head Roll (8-2)

❶ Start in the neutral supine position with your hands resting on your lower ribs.

❷ Inhale deeply. On the exhale, float your left arm straight up to the ceiling, keeping your shoulder girdle neutral. **(8-2a)**

❸ Inhale deeply. On the exhale, move your left shoulder blade out and away from your spine and reach your left arm closer to the ceiling, stretching your upper back muscles. Your left shoulder tip should move down and away from your left ear, not hunch up toward it. **(8-2b)**

❹ Inhale deeply, maintaining the stretch. Exhale, pull your left shoulder blade farther out and away, and reach your left arm farther toward the ceiling.

❺ Repeat the breathing/stretch sequence once more.

❻ Inhale deeply. On the exhale, release all muscular effort, allowing your left shoulder to drop to the floor; your left hand comes to rest on your lower ribs.

❼ Repeat on the other side.

❽ Keeping your head on the floor, rotate your head so that the back of your head moves farther away from your torso. Hold the rotation for a moment or two and then release all muscular effort. (Your head may rebound slightly.)

❾ Repeat the entire sequence once, left and right sides, with head rotation.

GOALS

→ Stretches the muscles of the upper back, neck, and rotator cuff.

→ Aligns the shoulder girdle.

→ Aligns the upper spine and head.

TRAINING TIPS

→ Your shoulder tip will tend to creep toward your ear as you slide your shoulder blade away from your spine. Focus on moving your shoulder tip down and away from your ear.

→ Keep your spine and rib cage absolutely stable as you stretch your arm.

→ If you are very flexible, take care that you do not over-flatten your neck on the head roll.

Exercise After Pregnancy: How to Look and Feel Your Best

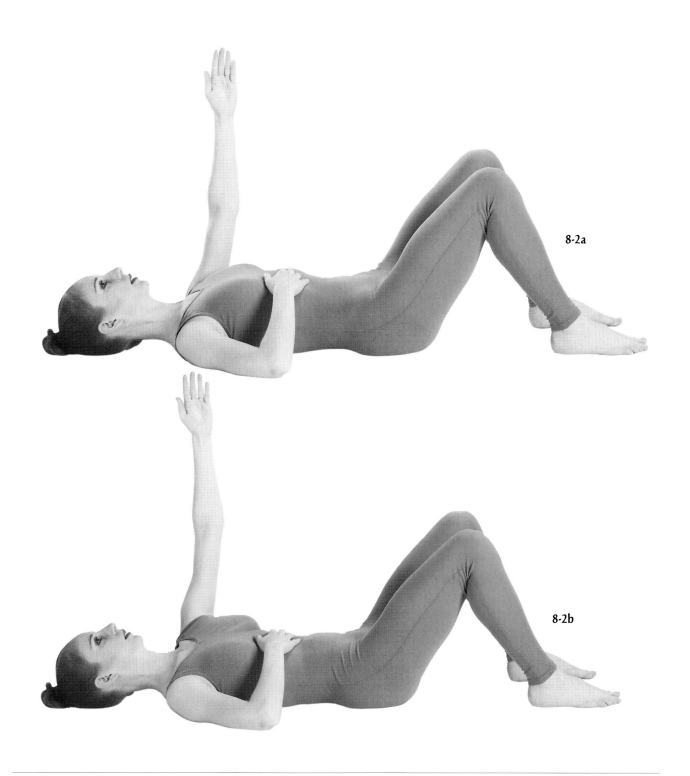

8-2a

8-2b

Isometric Pushes (8-3)

❶ Start in the hollow tuck position. Place both hands on your right thigh near your knee. Press your shoulder tips to the floor. Tighten your abdominal wall and close your pelvic floor.

❷ Firmly push your right leg away from your body with your hands as you simultaneously pull your knee toward your chest. Balance the opposing forces so that your thigh does not move. You will feel a strong isometric contraction in your hip flexors and lower abdominal wall. **(8-3)**

❸ Maintain the push of your arms for six seconds, then relax.

❹ Place your hands on your left thigh. Repeat on the left side.

❺ Perform five times on each side.

GOALS

➤ Strengthens the hip flexors.

➤ Flattens the abdominal wall.

➤ Strengthens the shoulder girdle.

TRAINING TIPS

➤ It is possible to generate a lot of force in this exercise. Take care that your abdominal wall remains tight and flat and that your pelvic floor stays closed.

➤ Push your shoulder blades firmly down your back to maintain good upper body alignment.

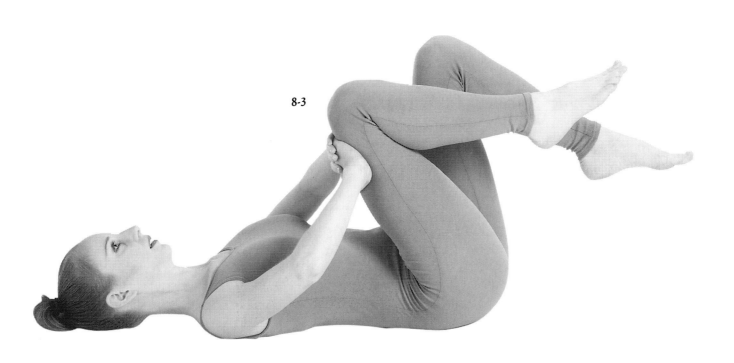

8-3

Alternating Toe Slides (8-4)

❶ Start in the hollow tuck position.

❷ Release your right leg, sliding your foot lightly along the floor until your leg is almost straight. Maintain the hollow pelvic tilt. **(8-4a)**

❸ Pull your right knee back into your chest (keeping your foot in contact with the floor for as long as possible) as your left leg releases and begins to extend along the floor. Your legs will function like a pulley, with one side extending as the other flexes. **(8-4b)**

❹ Start the slides at a slow tempo and gradually build up speed as you gain strength and control. As always, make sure that your pelvis and lower spine do not move and that your abdominal wall stays flat and pressed into your spine.

❺ Perform thirty-two repetitions or stop when your body fatigues.

GOALS

➥ Develops core strength.

➥ Strengthens the abdominal wall.

TRAINING TIPS

➥ Exchange your legs evenly so that both legs are constantly moving in opposition.

➥ To help center your body and develop dynamic stability, imagine that you are in a canoe; don't rock the boat as you perform the exercise.

➥ For an additional challenge, perform this exercise with your arms perpendicular to the floor, keeping your shoulder girdle neutral.

Exercise After Pregnancy: How to Look and Feel Your Best

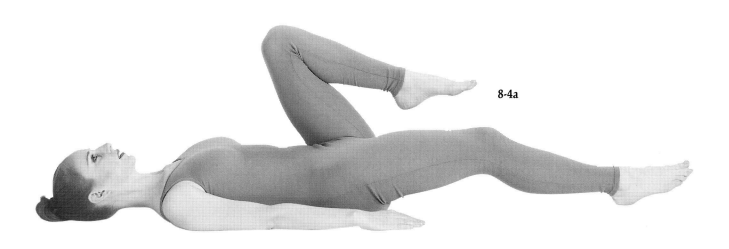

8-4a

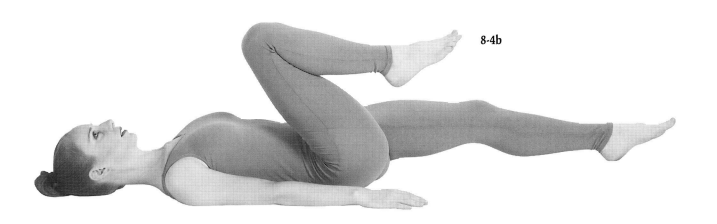

8-4b

Full Leg Arcs (8-5)

❶ Start in the hollow tuck position. Flex both feet. Straighten your right leg so that it is perpendicular to the floor. **(8-5a)**

❷ Slowly, in two counts, lower your right leg until your heel is just off the floor as you pull your left knee closer to your chest. As in the Small Leg Arcs **(7-5)**, take care that your pubic bone does not follow your right leg and that your abdominal wall stays flat and pressed into the spine. Keep your lower back firmly anchored to the floor. **(8-5b)**

❸ Bend your right knee and pull your thigh back to your chest. Reassert the hollow pelvic tilt.

❹ Lift your left leg perpendicular to the floor and repeat on the other side.

❺ Perform eight leg arcs on each side.

GOALS

➤ Develops core strength.

➤ Strengthens and flattens the abdominal wall.

➤ Develops dynamic stability.

TRAINING TIPS

➤ Take care that you don't start "bicycling" your legs. If you do, your quadriceps will take over most of the work.

➤ For an additional challenge, perform this exercise with your arms perpendicular to the floor.

Exercise After Pregnancy: How to Look and Feel Your Best

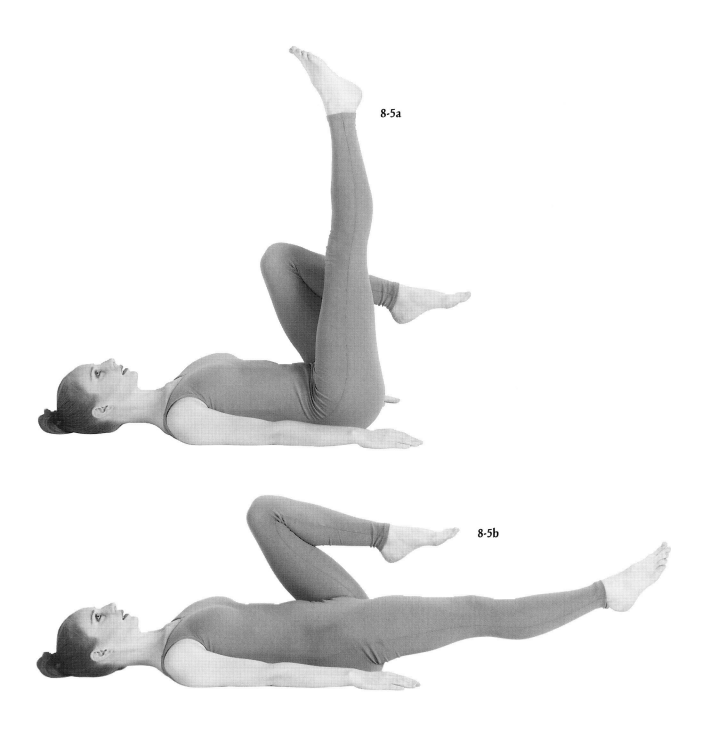

8-5a

8-5b

Leg Circles (8-6)

❶ Start in the hollow tuck position. Straighten both legs perpendicular to the floor. Draw your shoulder blades down your back, press your shoulder tips lightly to the floor, and lengthen the back of your neck. **(8-6a)**

❷ Start a circle by moving your right leg directly to the right side. **(8-6b)**

❸ Continue the circle by drawing your right leg around and down until your right heel is slightly off the floor. **(8-6c)**

❹ Lever your right leg straight back up to perpendicular. Keep both legs straight, left leg perpendicular to the floor throughout the exercise.

❺ Repeat with the left leg. Perform eight repetitions, alternating sides.

GOALS

- Strengthens the abdominal wall and develops core strength.

- Develops three-dimensional dynamic stability.

TRAINING TIPS

- This is a challenging exercise. Take care that your hips never wobble during your leg circle. Adjust the size of your circle so that you can maintain a stable position. Keep your chest open, your shoulders neutral, the back of your neck long, and your chin to your chest. As always, aim for precision and control. Increase your range of motion as you develop strength.

- For those who seek the ultimate challenge, perform this exercise with your arms perpendicular to the floor.

Exercise After Pregnancy: How to Look and Feel Your Best

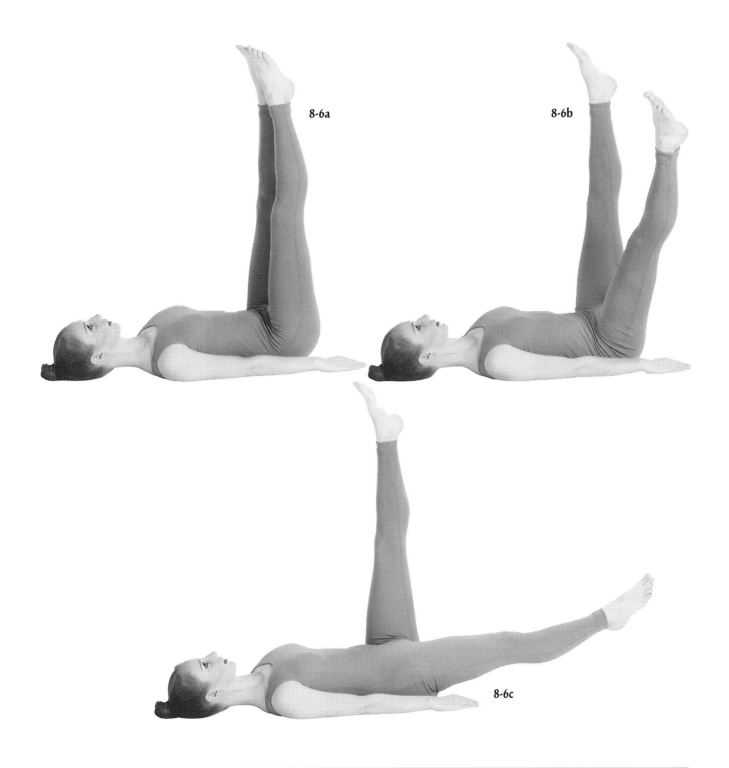

8-6a

8-6b

8-6c

Scissors (8-7)

❶ Start in the hollow tuck position. Straighten both legs perpendicular to the floor. Draw your shoulder blades down your back, press your shoulder tips lightly to the floor, and lengthen the back of your neck. **(8-7a)**

❷ In a slow two-count, open your legs to a wide "V." **(8-7b)**

❸ Close your legs in a slow two-count, drawing as long an arc with your legs as you can.

❹ Firmly cross the tops of your thighs and "scissor" your legs four times, alternating front and back. Keep legs straight throughout the sequence. (Knees will pass each other.) **(8-7c)**

❺ Perform six repetitions.

GOALS

➤ Strengthens the inner thighs and quadriceps.

➤ Strengthens the abdominal wall.

➤ Develops dynamic stability.

TRAINING TIPS

➤ Stretch your legs away from your torso throughout the exercise.

➤ Take care that your legs do not overpower your abdominal wall as your knees cross.

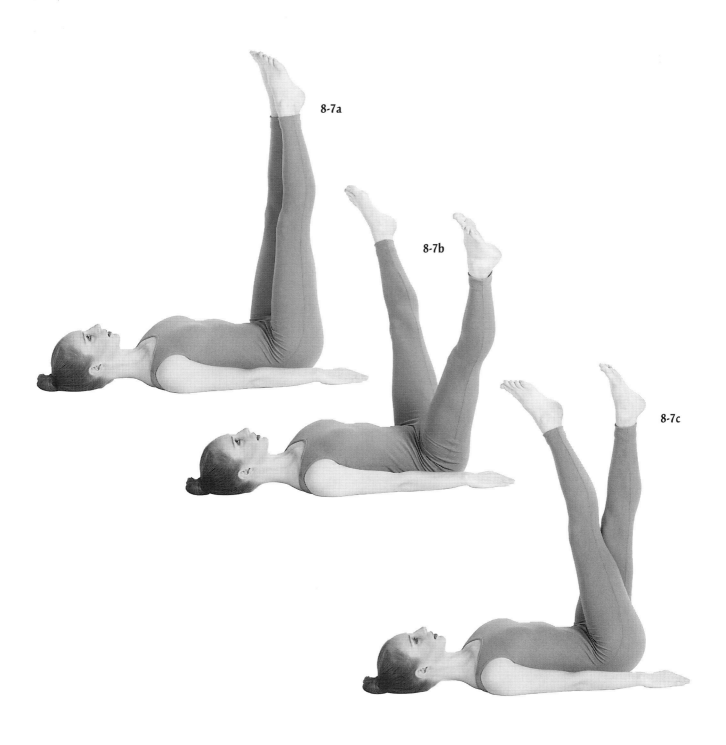

8-7a

8-7b

8-7c

Full Reverse Curls (8-8)

❶ Start in the hollow tuck position. Lift your legs to form a 90-degree angle, thighs perpendicular and shins parallel to the floor. **(8-8a)**

❷ Roll your lower spine off the floor by contracting your abdominals until your feet come over your hips. Hold the top of the curl for a moment. **(8-8b)**

❸ Roll down slowly.

❹ Tilt your legs slightly to the right, keeping both sides of your pelvis in contact with the floor. **(8-8c)**

❺ Roll your lower spine off the floor with your legs to the right side. Hold the top of the curl for a moment. **(8-8d)**

❻ Roll down slowly.

❼ Repeat center and left side.

❽ Perform eight sets (center, right, center, and left).

Strengthens the lower abdominal wall.

TRAINING TIPS

Keep your thighs fairly close to your chest. Curl your lower spine off the floor as if you were going to perform a backward somersault as opposed to a shoulder stand.

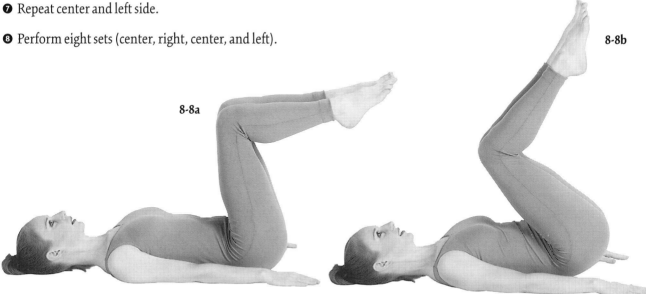

8-8a

8-8b

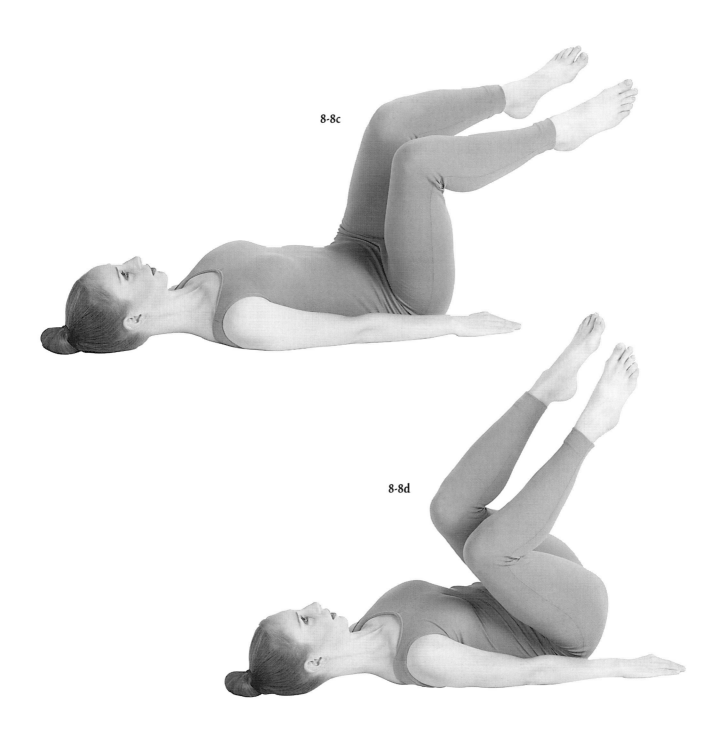

8-8c

8-8d

Twisters (8-9)

❶ Start in the hollow tuck position. Put both hands behind your head, shoulders down, elbows in your peripheral vision. Elongate the back of your neck using your hands to help support your head. **(8-9a)**

❷ Toe tap with your left foot as your upper body twists to the right. **(8-9b)**

❸ Reverse your leg and body positions. Keep your pelvis absolutely still. **(8-9c)**

❹ As you continue changing sides, increase your range of motion so that your legs slide out as far as you can control—as in the Alternating Toe Slides **(8-4)**.

❺ Try for sixteen repetitions (left and right) in one set. Rest for ten to fifteen seconds between sets. Perform three sets in all.

GOALS

→ Strengthens all four layers of the abdominal wall.

→ Strengthens the hip flexors.

→ Develops dynamic stability.

TRAINING TIPS

→ Do not perform this exercise if you have abdominal separation.

→ This is a very challenging exercise, and your body will fatigue quickly. Maintain good form. Rest whenever necessary.

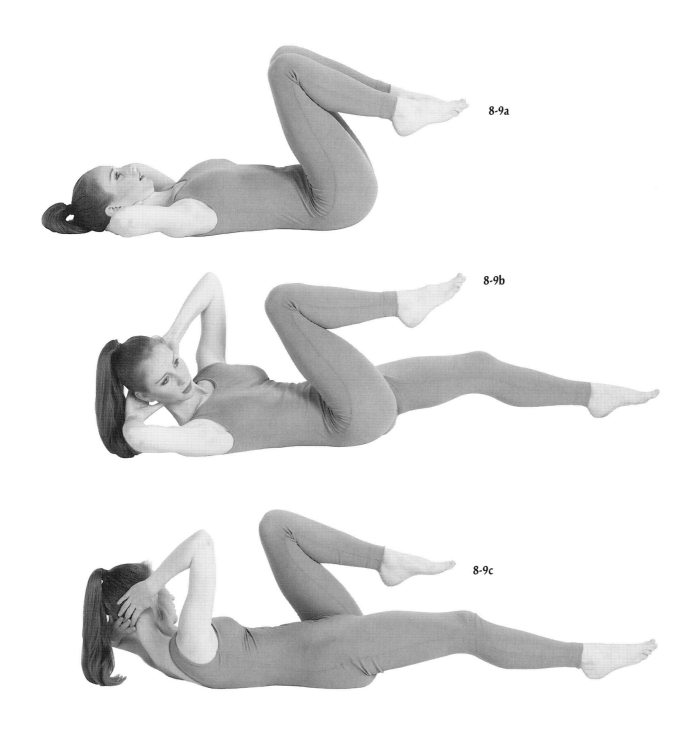

8-9a

8-9b

8-9c

The Egg (8-10)

❶ Start in the hollow tuck position. Roll your upper spine off the floor (an upper body crunch) as you reach your arms past your hips. Keep your shoulders wide and down your back. Pull your knees in as far as you can, so that you make your tightest "egg." **(8-10a)**

❷ Roll your upper body down to the neutral position (ribs down, back of your neck long) as you lift your arms to a diagonal above your head and extend your legs to a low diagonal. Your palms face each other and stay twelve to sixteen inches apart, hands in your peripheral vision. **(8-10b)**

❸ Circle your arms to the side, around, and down as your legs bend, and pull your thighs firmly into your chest as your upper body curves back up into the egg position. Keep your shoulders wide and down your back.

❹ Perform eight repetitions.

GOALS

➠ Strengthens all four layers of the abdominal wall.

➠ Develops dynamic stability.

➠ Integrates the lower and upper spine.

TRAINING TIPS

Anchor your pelvis, rib cage, and head in the neutral position on the floor in one movement as you firmly extend your limbs. Make sure that your ribs don't flare open and that your spine does not hyperextend.

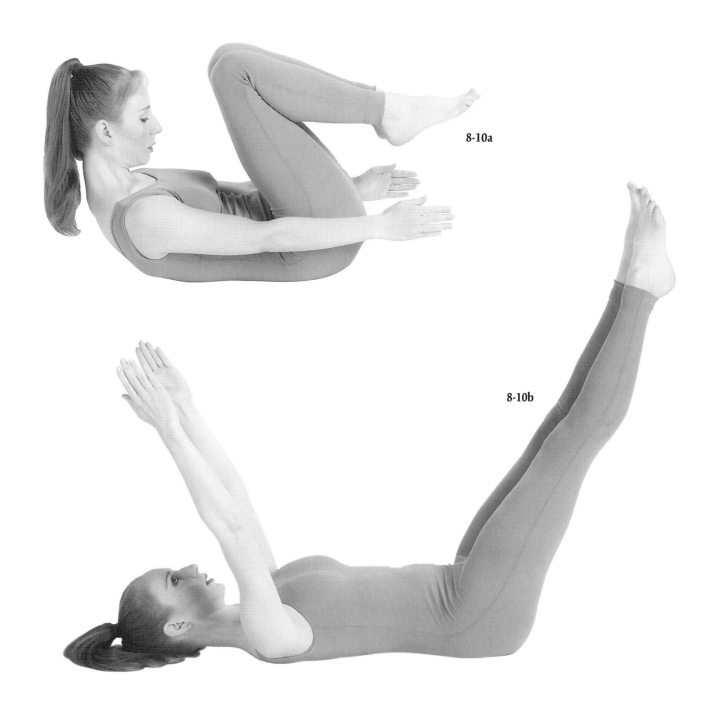

8-10a

8-10b

Superwoman (8-11)

❶ Lie prone, forehead on the floor, legs close together, feet extended. Place your hands by your shoulders, your elbows close to your waist.

❷ Using your abdominal wall (no gluteals), perform a hollow pelvic tilt. Your belly will lift off the floor (or try to) and your pubic bone will anchor to the floor. **(8-11a)**

❸ Lift your head two inches off the floor.

❹ Lift your chest slightly off the floor without using your arms. Slide your shoulder blades down your back and slightly together. **(8-11b)**

❺ Reach both arms forward so that they are in line with your head, palms facing down, twelve to sixteen inches apart. **(8-11c)**

❻ Stretch your legs and lift them about six inches off the floor (the gluteals will work here). Hold the position for four seconds. **(8-11d)**

❼ Lengthen your spine as you release back into the starting position. Perform eight repetitions.

GOALS

➥ Strengthens the upper back.

➥ Strengthens the lower back.

➥ Strengthens the gluteals.

➥ Stabilizes the lower spine.

TRAINING TIPS

➥ Maintain a strong hollow pelvic tilt so that your lower back does not arch. If you feel any compression in your lower back, you've gone too far.

➥ If you have recurring lower back problems, keep your legs on the floor.

➥ If your body needs it, release the spine in Child's Pose **(7-12)** after this exercise.

Exercise After Pregnancy: How to Look and Feel Your Best

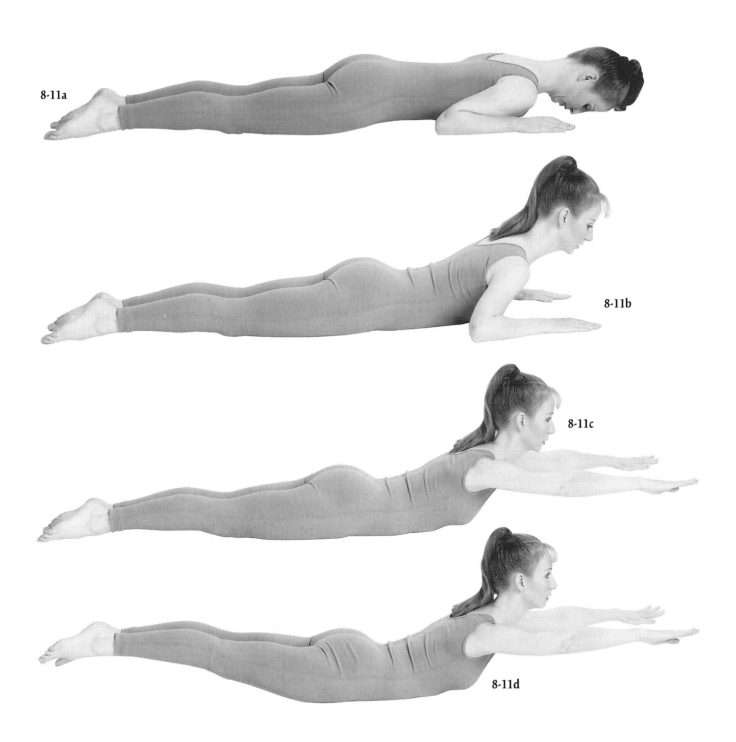

8-11a

8-11b

8-11c

8-11d

A-Frame Pushups (8-12)

❶ Start in the quadruped position. Straighten your legs and push your tailbone up toward the ceiling to form an "A." Lift your abdominal wall toward your spine as much as you can. **(8-12a)**

❷ Bend your arms (elbows move to each side) to lower your upper body; the top of your head will almost touch the floor between your hands. (Go only as far as you can and maintain control.) Keep your spine neutral, shoulders pressed down, legs straight, abdominals tight. **(8-12b)**

❸ Push back up into the starting position.

❹ Perform ten repetitions.

GOALS

Strengthens the upper back, shoulders, and arms.

TRAINING TIPS

Maintain the triangle shape of your body as you bend your arms so that the top of your head stays in line with your hands. You don't want to move your upper body forward into a standard pushup position.

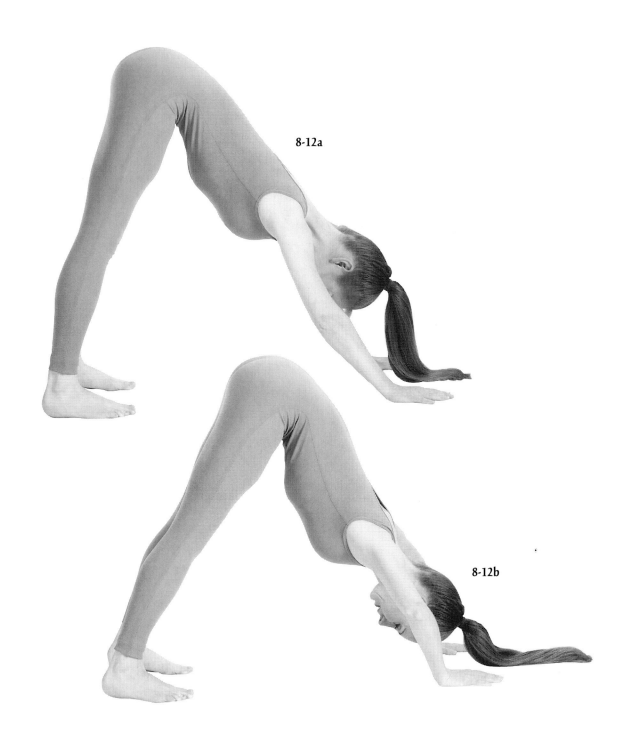

8-12a

8-12b

Deep Squats
with Elbow Pulses (8-13)

❶ Stand tall, pelvis neutral, spine long, feet slightly wider than the hips (parallel second), and arms extended straight up. **(8-13a)**

❷ Simultaneously bend your hips, knees, and ankles, moving your spine to a high diagonal. (Keep your spine neutral, your lumbar curve intact.)

❸ Start the pulses by deepening the bend of your knees as you bend your arms and bring your elbows to your waist, forearms parallel to each other. (Your shoulder blades will move down and slightly together.) **(8-13b)**

❹ Pulse your legs and arms in unison. Keep your knees over your feet, your arches intact.

❺ Continue pulsing until your body begins to fatigue; then rise back to the starting position—pelvis neutral, spine long and supported by the abdominal wall, arms extended overhead.

❻ Repeat the squat/pulse sequence twice.

GOALS

➤ Strengthens the spine, upper back, abdominals, hips, and legs.

➤ Prepares the body for ergonomic lifting.

TRAINING TIPS

➤ Start with the number of pulses you can do while maintaining good form. Slowly add a few pulses each time until you can do thirty-two in a row.

➤ Make sure your shoulder blades don't hunch up as you fatigue.

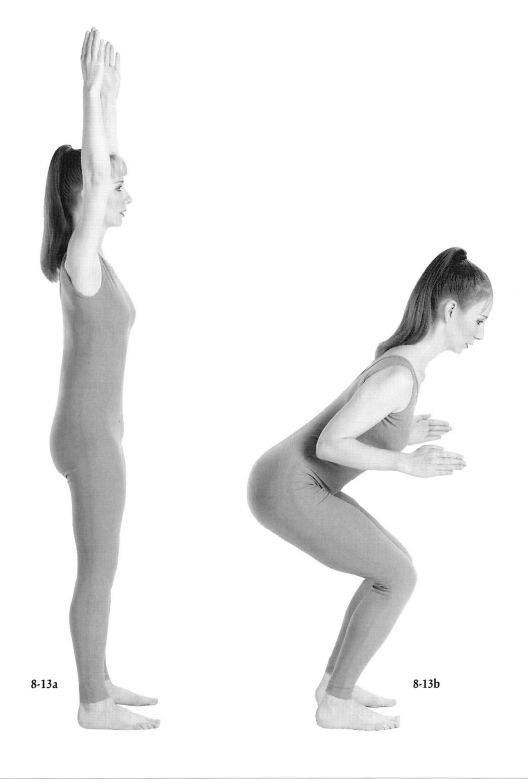

8-13a

8-13b

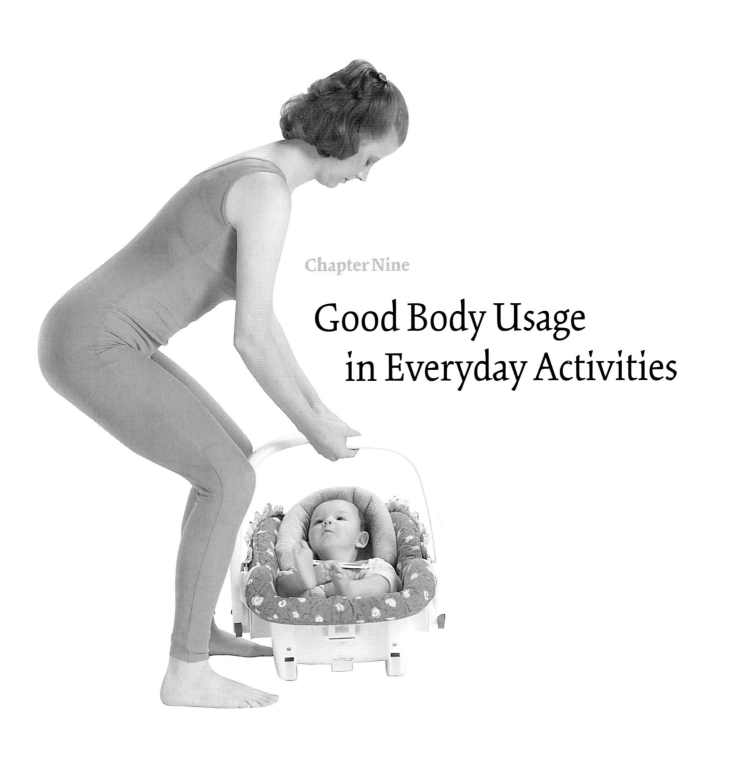

Chapter Nine

Good Body Usage
in Everyday Activities

"As I bent down to pick up a pencil from the floor, my back suddenly went into a spasm and I couldn't move!" As a personal trainer, I've heard many stories like this one. Like the proverbial straw that breaks the camel's back, it is all too common for our backs to "go out" during a mundane and seemingly inconsequential movement. Of course it's not the weight of the pencil that brings on a spasm, but the years of poor body usage that finally take their toll.

The spine is more vulnerable to injury after pregnancy. Because of instability and altered alignment, good body usage in everyday activities—lifting, carrying, and nursing—is essential. It greatly reduces wear and tear on joints, ligaments, and muscles; reduces the potential for injury, and helps eliminate painful spasms.

Ironically, when we are at our structural weakest, we are called upon to lift and carry our newborns almost constantly. No wonder so many new mothers complain of lower back pain, midback pain, shoulder spasms, and neck pain. As we have seen, the spine and pelvis are out of ideal alignment after childbirth. When the bones are out of alignment, the entire neuromuscular system functions poorly, which in turn increases the load on muscles, ligaments, and articular surfaces of joints, particularly the vertebral discs. These stresses accumulate until even the smallest movement can trigger a painful spasm.

We've all heard the mantra "Lift with the legs," but in order to take advantage of the power muscles of the legs and hips, the spine must be properly aligned and stabilized in the neutral position. And that means we must squat (bending only the hips, knees, and ankles) rather than stoop (curving the spine) when we lift. When we stoop and lift, the back muscles cannot help support the spine, regardless of whether the knees are flexed or straight. Because stooping is general-ly aligned with the force of gravity, it is too easy to collapse the upper body and neglect to tighten the abdominal wall.

In contrast, squatting allows the spine to function as an integrated unit, with the load evenly distributed throughout the body. No single area bears the brunt of the work. During a squat, the back muscles and the abdominals co-contract isometrically to create a dynamic cylinder of support for the torso. The spine functions as one long lever. And, of course, the longer the lever, the stronger it is.

For many women, squatting while maintaining a neutral spine is not easy. They have been conditioned to be "lady-like," which means not allowing their backsides to protrude when they bend to pick up something. As a result, they have weak back muscles. Other women have been instructed in aerobics or fitness classes to make a flat back by slightly tucking the tailbone under or by pushing the waistline back during squats, lunges, or exercises on all fours. Many people mistakenly believe they are protecting their backs when they flatten their lumbar curve. But when the lumbar curve is flattened, the long muscles of the back cannot contract to help create a dynamic core that supports and stabilizes the spine.

The time to learn good body usage is now, while your baby is small and relatively light. As your baby grows, you will have the skills and strength to deal with the ever-increasing load.

The golden rule for lifting and carrying is to align and stabilize your spine and shoulder girdle before you begin the physical task.

Principles of Lifting (9-1)

❶ Directly face the object you want to lift—square off. Your legs are parallel (knees facing forward). Your feet are slightly farther apart than the width of your hips and can be opposite each other (second position) or in the step position with one foot slightly in front of the other (fourth position). Some women, especially those with wide hips, find a slight outward rotation of the legs and feet to be more natural. If you use this stance, be sure your knees track directly over your feet, your shins remain perpendicular to the floor, and the arches of your feet are intact.

❷ Align your spine in the neutral position. Firmly pull your abdominal wall in toward your spine. Press your shoulder blades down your back and slightly together. Push the back of your head back and up so that your ears align over your shoulders.

❸ Squat directly over the object you want to lift by simultaneously bending your hips, knees, and ankles. Your spine will move to a high diagonal. Lower yourself by bending your knees deeply. You want to be directly above and as close to the object as possible without curving your spine or rolling your ankles in. Keep your lower legs perpendicular to the floor, knees over your feet. **(9-1a)**

❹ Lift the object straight up and into your body. You want the lifting action to be as close to vertical as possible. **(9-1b)**

❺ Push through your legs and return your spine to an upright position. Keep your abdominals tight and your shoulders pressed down your back. **(9-1c)** After pregnancy, many women tend to release the abdominals (allowing the spine to hyperextend) and to hunch up the shoulders when lifting.

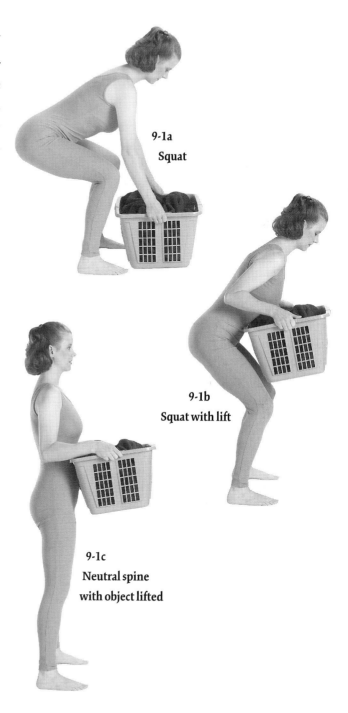

9-1a
Squat

9-1b
Squat with lift

9-1c
Neutral spine
with object lifted

To set an object on the floor, reverse the process. Be sure to complete the squat before extending your arms. Don't try to reach out and down; you want the object to move in a direct line with gravity.

Getting things like groceries and strollers out of the backseat or trunk of a car presents a common ergonomic problem. Many of us reach out with a curved spine and try to lift the object while it is far from our bodies. Instead, drag the object as close to your body as possible before lifting.

To lift your baby off the floor, kneel beside her and flex deeply through the hips with your spine on a diagonal, mimicking the squat position. Stabilize and support your spine using the same techniques you would during a squat. Pick up your baby and hold her close before you try to stand. Place one foot adjacent to your opposite knee so that you have a 90-degree angle at both your hip and knee joints. This creates a wide base of support, which increases stability. Put one hand on a piece of furniture or a wall for balance. Push through the legs to stand.

Carrying (9-2)

Once you have lifted your baby (or another load), it is important to maintain a supported spine. Keep your pelvis neutral, abdominals tight, shoulders down your back, ears aligned over the shoulders, and spine long. Many women mistakenly hollow out their chest when carrying their babies, which stresses the upper spine. While carrying your baby, try to pull your body weight out of your lower back.

Most baby frontpacks are problematic. The shoulders and upper back muscles must constantly work to keep the body upright and support the weight of the baby. After pregnancy, these muscles are already working too hard; the added load exacerbates the problem, increasing upper back stiffness and poor alignment of the shoulder girdle and upper spine.

Frontpacks place your baby in a very similar position as during pregnancy. But because the postpartum body lacks abdominal control, it is almost impossible to keep the pelvis from tipping, the chest from collapsing, and the head from sliding forward—exactly what we want to counterbalance, especially when we exercise.

Baby slings have advantages and disadvantages. On the plus side, most of them have wide shoulder straps that help disperse the load. However, they place an asymmetrical load on the body, causing more strain. When you use a sling, one shoulder and the opposite side of your lower back constantly work to maintain an upright position.

If you decide to use a sling, alternate sides every time. This will feel awkward at first, and your nondominant side will have to get used to it. But in the long run, alternating sides is by far the best solution.

Whenever possible, put your baby in a stroller instead of a frontpack. Many women push their babies around the house while they attend to older children, fix meals, and so on. When your baby has good head control, by about six months, an ergonomic backpack that is sized for your spine and has a hip belt is great for fitness walking and chores around the house.

As your baby grows into a toddler and can wrap her legs around your waist to help hold on, you may be tempted to thrust one hip out for her to sit on. This asymmetrical posture strains muscles, ligaments, and vertebral discs. When your toddler is a little older, you may choose to squat deeply and have her climb on so you can carry her on your back (with your hands interlocked behind your back, under her bottom). This position places your child's weight directly over your center of gravity; you can carry your child safely this way for a long time.

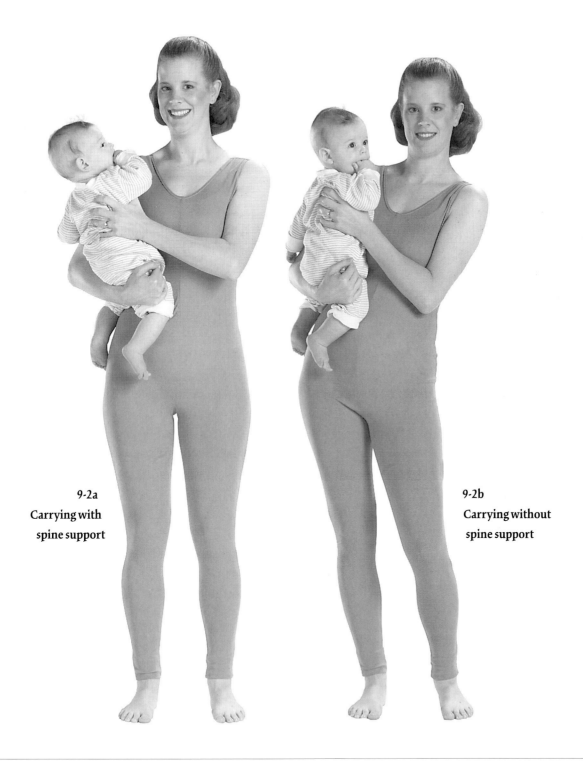

9-2a
Carrying with
spine support

9-2b
Carrying without
spine support

Car Seats (9-3)

To get your baby in and out of the car seat, lower the handle so that the baby can be placed directly in. Put the car seat on a table, bed, or sturdy chair so that you're not tempted to stoop to the floor. Lifting the car seat with your baby in it is much easier if the seat is already elevated. Of course, you never want to leave your baby unattended—even for a moment—in a car seat that is not on the floor. The use of a table, chair, or bed is appropriate only while you are getting your baby in and out of the seat.

Putting the car seat into its base is always awkward. Break the movements into small, controlled motions. Don't simultaneously lunge and reach, trying to accomplish the physical action in one movement; it's much too hard on your back.

❶ Start with the car door open and your baby in the car seat on the ground as close to you as possible. Squat and lift the car seat using the techniques described in Principles of Lifting **(9-1)**. Be careful not to twist and lift at the same time.

❷ Place one foot on the lower edge of the door frame. Shift your weight forward and onto that foot as you put your baby on the backseat.

❸ If you are small enough or have a large enough vehicle, get into your car opposite your baby. Move the front seats all the way forward to gain the maximum space. Squat, and lift the car seat. Transfer your weight laterally toward the seat base as you place the seat onto the base. You want to avoid reaching out. Transferring your body weight in the direction you move your baby will help reduce stress on your back. If you cannot fit entirely in the backseat area, get as much of your body (particularly your pelvis) in the car as possible. Try to keep your spine as close to neutral as possible.

❹ Adjust the seat in the base so that it locks securely.

To get your baby and car seat out, reverse the action. Remember, it is safer to do small, controlled movements, shifting your body position to gain leverage, than it is to reach over, unlock, and lift up and out in one action.

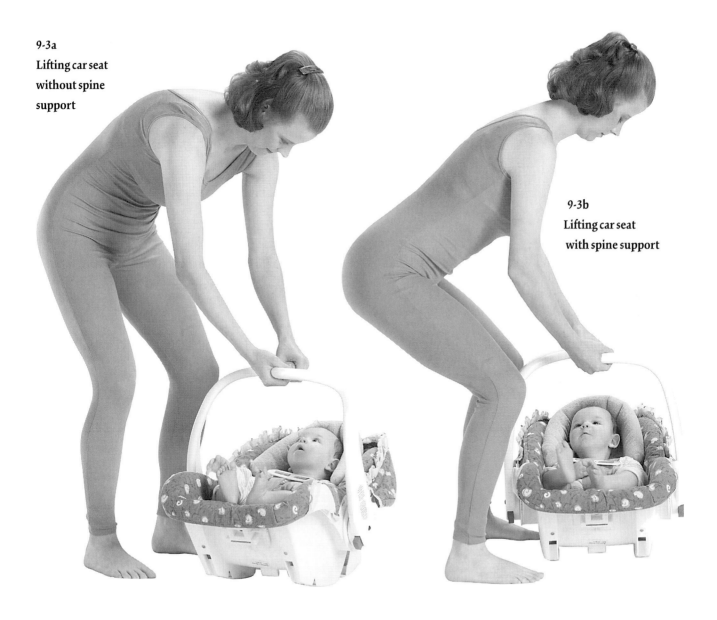

9-3a
Lifting car seat
without spine
support

9-3b
Lifting car seat
with spine support

Sitting and Breast-Feeding Positions (9-4)

New mothers spend many hours a day breast-feeding and/or bottle-feeding their babies. Give your back a break by setting up a breast-feeding station in your house, with a good chair and pillows to ensure that your spine and shoulders are in the best position possible. Many couches and chairs are designed for style, not ergonomics. When it comes to furniture, one size definitely does not fit all.

In the ideal sitting position **(9-4a)**, your feet rest flat on the floor with a right angle at both your knees and hips. Your pelvis and spine should be neutral. Your body weight will be on the bottom of your pelvis (the ischium), not rolled back on your tailbone or sacroiliac joint (the back of your pelvis) **(9-4b)**.

Most chairs and couches offer no support to the lower back. It is almost impossible to sit in one without rolling back off the pelvis, curving the spine, and hunching the shoulders. Sitting with poor posture places more stress on the ligaments and the vertebral disks than standing poorly does. Lumbar support pillows, which allow the spine to relax in the neutral position, are great to use when you're sitting. You can also roll a hand towel into a cylinder and place it behind the small of your back.

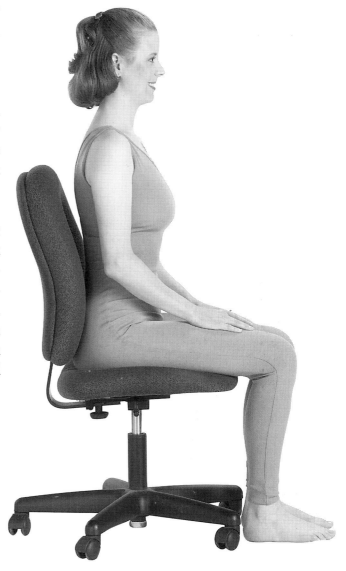

9-4a
Sitting with neutral spine

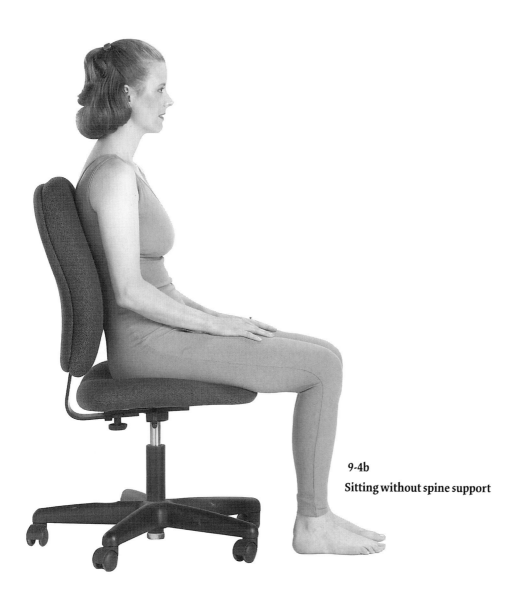

9-4b

Sitting without spine support

Since the lumbar curve is determined by the angle of the pelvis, it is important to maintain a vertical bikini triangle while sitting. If the seat length is too long in proportion to the length of your thighs (as it often is, if you are on the small side), you will also need to stuff a pillow behind your pelvis to fill the gap.

Many women tend to bring their breasts down to their baby during nursing, rather than bringing their baby up to their breasts. **(9-4d)** This curves the upper back, rolls the shoulders in, shortens the muscles on the front of the chest, and is a primary cause of upper back pain and shoulder spasms. Depending on your body proportions, you may need two or more pillows on your lap so that your spine can be in the neutral position when nursing. **(9-4c)**

Try to relax your shoulders so that they fall naturally down your back. Align your head so that your ears are directly over your shoulders.

Ideally, your baby is well balanced and at a height where you do not need to constantly use your arms or hands to support her while feeding.

Many large-breasted women feel that they must lift and support the nipple with one hand while nursing. This position places a lot of strain on the wrist. In most cases, the nipple hangs at a poor angle because the mother's shoulders and upper back are rounded. When the spine is in the neutral position, the nipple automatically lifts to an advantageous angle for feeding. Because carpal tunnel syndrome and other repetitive stress injuries commonly occur during and after pregnancy, holding the breast while feeding is a particularly risky habit.

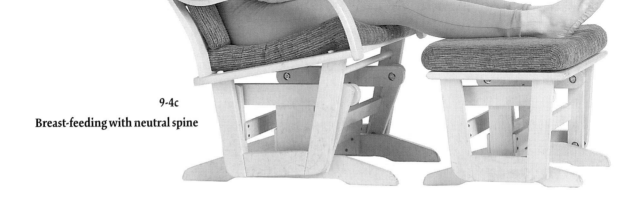

9-4c
Breast-feeding with neutral spine

Exercise After Pregnancy: How to Look and Feel Your Best

Another common mistake is to cross the legs at the knees or to place one ankle across the opposite knee to raise the baby higher. Both positions stretch ligaments in the lower back, further reducing the stability of the sacroiliac joint. Keep your feet flat on the floor or on a footstool. Use an extra pillow to elevate your baby if necessary.

Many women choose to nurse their babies while lying in bed, especially during nighttime feedings. Again, avoid hunching down to your baby's mouth. Either raise your baby in the bed or lower your body so that your spine can be neutral. When you lie on your side, try to keep your hips stacked over each other so that your spine does not twist. Many women find that a pillow stuffed behind the pelvis and waist area offers extra support.

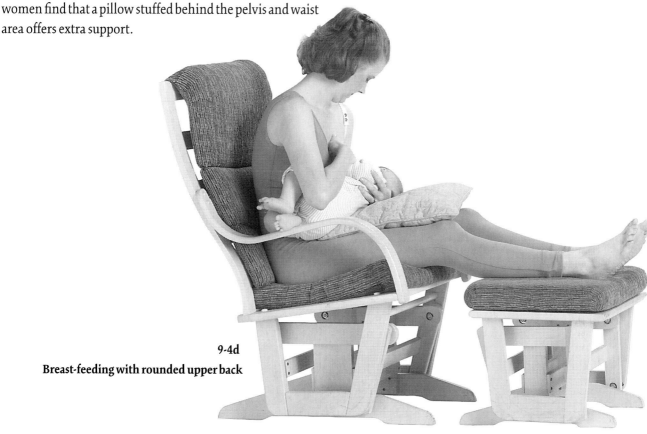

9-4d
Breast-feeding with rounded upper back

Carpal tunnel syndrome (CTS) occurs when the median nerve, which supplies sensation to most of the hand and fingers, is compressed as it passes through the wrist and into the hand. CTS can be one side effect of pregnancy. Fluid retention and swelling caused by hormonal changes can put pressure on the median nerve and neighboring tendons. In most cases, CTS resolves on its own after pregnancy, but some women continue to experience symptoms. For these women, the daily activities of baby care can worsen symptoms dramatically. Because CTS and related repetitive stress injuries can lead to chronic, debilitating pain, never ignore symptoms such as pain, tingling, numbness, or weakness in your wrists and hands. Consult your doctor and get a referral to a physical therapist specializing in repetitive stress injuries. Here are two tests for CTS. If you feel pain in the inverted prayer position or when you tap lightly on the base of your hand, you may have a repetitive stress injury.

Practicing good ergonomics can be frustrating at first. Most people find themselves unconsciously slipping into old habits and correcting their postures throughout the day. This is normal. But the more you are conscious of good movement patterns, the quicker they will become unconscious habits.

9-5a
Carpal tunnel test: inverted prayer position. Put the backs of your hands together, fingers facing down, in front of your chest.

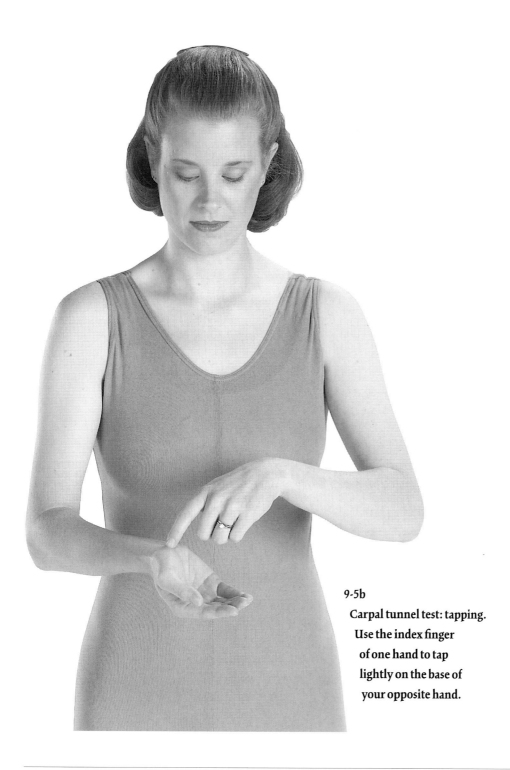

9-5b
Carpal tunnel test: tapping.
Use the index finger
of one hand to tap
lightly on the base of
your opposite hand.

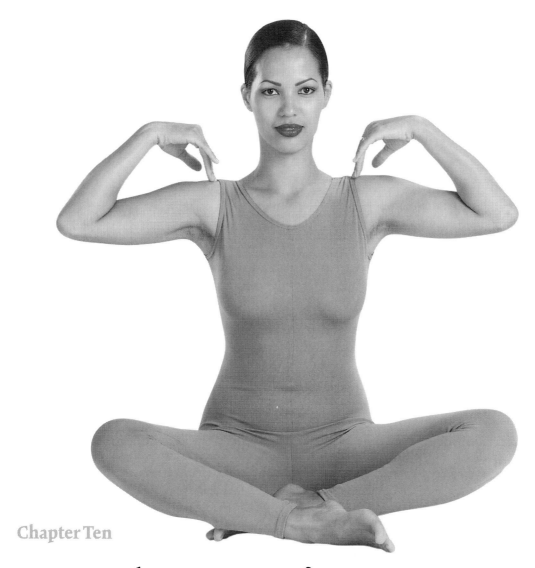

Chapter Ten

Body Image After Pregnancy

Sore nipples, hemorrhoids, urinary incontinence, episiotomy pain, anal fissures, cesarean incision pain, vaginal dryness, sleep deprivation—these are just some of the physical aggravations women face after pregnancy. Then there's body image, perhaps the most difficult issue of all. It's a sensitive and complex topic, one that is often hard for women to talk about. We're supposed to be basking in the joys of new motherhood, not worrying (stupidly? selfishly?) about our figures.

Body image and self-acceptance are hard to grapple with even in the best of times. New motherhood is a period of heightened stress as we adapt to the changes a new baby brings. For many, psychological stress can be like a funhouse mirror, warping our view of ourselves and exacerbating body image problems. We live in a culture where having a "mommy body" has never been more of a challenge. The importance of beauty, youth, and extreme thinness, along with unrealistic, unhealthy expectations about what the female form should look like, sets up a no-win situation for most women.

Being heavier than your prepregnancy weight and having a round, soft belly, stretch marks, and a closet full of clothes many sizes too small is difficult enough. But it is the deeper psychological issues that gnaw away at our sense of self-worth. We ask ourselves, "Will I ever get my body back?" "Will I ever fit into my clothes?" "Is this the beginning of the end for my body (and therefore my youth)?" And perhaps most crucially, "Am I still sexually desirable to my mate?"

I have found that the key to self-acceptance is to understand individual body types and to set appropriate and attainable goals that are based upon them. When a woman realizes that many aspects of her body are a reflection of her genetic makeup and that little can be done to alter them, a great burden is lifted. For many, the door to self-acceptance is finally unlocked.

Body types fall into three general classifications: the ectomorph, the mesomorph, and the endomorph. Most people display an overall dominance in one type with secondary characteristics in another. Each body type has strengths and weaknesses, and no type is inherently better than another.

The ectomorph has long thin bones and muscles. The hips, in women, tend to be wider than the shoulders. This body type has long ligaments and is loosely strung together. The ectomorph is naturally more flexible than the mesomorph or endomorph and can excel in activities such as ballet and yoga. But the ectomorph must work harder at strength and cardiovascular activities to achieve optimum functional balance and health. Because of their inherent elasticity, ectomorphs have less dynamic stability and are more vulnerable to joint injuries, osteoarthritis, and osteoporosis.

Ectomorphs have the fastest and most sensitive nervous system, which gives them a lower pain threshold. Ectomorphs are most likely to "carry" psychological stress in the body—for example, chronically tight shoulder muscles in response to stress. Because of the faster nervous system, ectomorphs digest food quickly and therefore take in proportionally fewer nutrients. This helps them stay slim. As you have probably guessed, the ectomorphic body type is fashionable. Since Twiggy took the world by storm in the 1960s, the vast majority of professional models have been extreme ectomorphs. Famous ectomorphs include Audrey Hepburn, Katharine Hepburn, and Gwyneth Paltrow.

The mesomorph has proportionally thicker, heavier

bones and muscles. The shoulders are as wide or wider than the hips, giving mesomorphs a more square look. Women with more extreme mesomorphic tendencies have noticeable muscularity even if they don't do strength-training activities. These bodies are built for strength, speed, and power. Mesomorphs utilize oxygen well and excel at aerobics and sports. Because they have tighter muscles and connective tissue, they are the least naturally flexible and must stretch diligently to achieve functional balance and reduce their vulnerability to muscle tears and pulls. Famous mesomorphs include Jackie Joyner-Kersee, Angela Bassett, and fitness pioneer Corey Everson.

The endomorph has soft, rounded body contours and a natural tendency to carry proportionally more body fat, which is fairly evenly distributed. This is the Rubenesque body type. Because bone density and ligament length tend to be moderate, the endomorph is the least vulnerable to sprains and muscle tears. Endomorphs have a slightly slower nervous system, and it is thought that the slower and more efficient digestive system contributes to the propensity to store fat, especially in women. Endomorphs can boost their metabolisms and keep a healthy body weight through a combination of regular aerobic activity, which utilizes stored fat as fuel, and strength training, which increases lean mass and raises basal metabolism. Throughout history, endomorphic women have been considered the most beautiful and desirable. Famous endomorphs include Mae West, Jane Russell, and Marilyn Monroe.

Many women mistakenly assume that they are endomorphic because they have a history of being, or perceiving themselves as, overweight. While obesity is a growing epidemic for children and adults, most women are not extreme endomorphs. Obesity is due to a combination of genetics, nutritional choices, and lifestyle choices—our dependence on highly processed grains, fast foods, and saturated fats; excessive sugar and calorie intake; extreme low-calorie diets; dangerous fad diets, and lack of physical activity. Ironically, many in our society are both overfed and undernourished.

That said, women's bodies are designed to carry a lot of stored fuel. The ideal percentage of body fat in the adult female is twenty to twenty-four percent. Professional and serious athletes often carry fifteen to twenty percent body fat. When you think about it, that's a lot of potential fuel. The extra fat stores we lay down in the last trimester of pregnancy are like an insurance policy; no matter what we might face—drought, fire, flood, famine—we will be able to grow and feed a healthy baby.

This is just one of the many ways Mother Nature stacks the odds in your baby's favor. So you gained weight during pregnancy? Congratulate yourself—your body did the right thing. Remember, most of your additional body weight after childbirth is not fat tissue. The average weight gain during pregnancy is twenty-five to thirty-five pounds, but only one-fifth, or four to six pounds, is extra fat storage.

Most postpartum women find themselves about fifteen pounds over their prepregnancy weight. That means only one-third of the extra weight is attributable to stored fat; the rest is comprised of fluids and the infrastructure needed to operate a 24-hour-a-day milk factory. It takes more energy to produce breast milk (about 500 extra calories a day) than to grow a baby (about 300 calories a day by the last trimester).

An average-size woman's basal metabolism requires about 2,000 calories a day. The additional 500 calories for lactation represents a twenty-five percent increase in needed fuel. This is why most nursing mothers feel ravenously hungry, especially after nursing.

In addition to increased calories, they need protein, calcium, vitamin D (for calcium absorption), and water. Many women have difficulty maintaining adequate hydration. Thirst is not a reliable indicator of hydration. Aim for an extra forty-eight ounces of water a day while you are nursing. Caffeinated drinks are diuretics and should be counted as a negative fluid, not a hydrator.

Dieting, or being calorie deficient, is particularly dangerous after pregnancy. It is unhealthy for both you and your baby. First, a calorie-deficient diet forces the body to burn both stored fat and muscle tissue. The ratio of fat to protein is generally about fifty-fifty. So when you go on a diet and lose twelve pounds, on average you will lose two pounds of fluids (exacerbating hydration problems), five pounds of fat, and five pounds of lean tissue. The loss of lean tissue lowers your basal metabolism, and you need even fewer calories to maintain your body weight. As you continue dieting, more lean tissue is lost, further lowering basal metabolism. As you can see, a downward spiral begins. When the diet is stopped, weight gain is almost inevitable.

The only safe way to lose fat and maintain muscle mass is to eliminate excessive calorie intake and burn the excess fat off through exercise. Weight loss through exercise can seem agonizingly slow, but it is permanent, and because you gain muscle mass, your metabolism is higher. Continued weight loss through exercise is that much easier to accomplish. This is why people who are in great shape can eat proportionally more food and not gain weight.

The secondary effects of a calorie-deficient diet can be very serious. Dieting leads to extreme physical fatigue—the last thing a new mother needs when she is sleep deprived to begin with. In addition, it is almost impossible to take in the recommended levels of vitamins and minerals while dieting. The body will "cannibalize" its resources, drawing minerals out of the bones in the production of breast milk and thereby increasing the risk of developing osteoporosis.

Because lactation requires more calories, dieting sets up conflicting impulses. The appetite centers in the brain tell you to eat, while the intellect says no, don't eat, you need to lose weight. This dichotomy makes us obsessive about food and deprives us of the natural pleasures it provides. Dieting increases anxiety and, when coupled with fatigue, can lead to depression.

Dieting also weakens the immune system, leaving you and your baby (if you are breast-feeding) more vulnerable to viruses and bacterial infections. The bottom line is don't diet! Instead, increase your family's nutritional health by eating lots of whole grains, fresh fruits and vegetables, legumes, and low-fat protein and calcium sources.

Contrary to popular belief, nursing mothers do not automatically lose their pregnancy fat stores faster than those who bottle-feed their babies. When you are nursing, your body wants to keep the pantry well stocked for your baby, who is dependent on your milk supply. Many women find that when they resume menstruation and their baby is getting substantial calories from solid foods, their bodies begin to let go of their extra reserves. Menstruation is the signal that your body is finished with pregnancy and that you are ready (at least in a biological sense) to get pregnant again.

Over the years of teaching postpartum exercise I have encountered just five or six students who return to their prepregnancy weight in three or four months. How your body responds to pregnancy, how much weight you are likely to gain (if you eat an appropriate amount), and how quickly your body rebounds from pregnancy are all influenced by your genetic makeup. Because these variables are mostly out of your control, it only makes sense to accept and embrace the inherent wisdom of your body. Focus on health-enhancing activities that are under your control: exercise and nutrition. It's the way to a better life.

Chapter Eleven

How to Achieve Your Goals

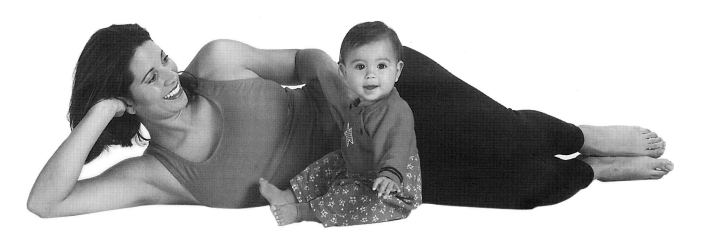

"I WANT TO LOSE WEIGHT." "I want to have a healthier lifestyle." "I want to look better in my clothes." This is typically how we state our health and fitness goals. And while these goals are admirable, they can be almost impossible to achieve. Why? Because they are multifaceted, end-result goals. Underlying each are numerous, more specific goals that must be reached first.

How we define our goals, or how we neglect to define them, sets the stage for success or failure. We all know the adage "A journey of a thousand miles starts with one step." In health and fitness, the compilation of many steps over time leads to success.

Take weight loss. Many nutrition issues must be analyzed to determine the steps that will maximize health and result in weight loss. In addition, specific fitness goals must be analyzed. Cardiovascular condition, strength assessment, flexibility, lean-mass ratio, and risk factors must be assessed. Further complicating the situation are the psychological issues that influence food choices and sometimes derail the best intentions.

Take the time to fully consider your goals. Write them down. Work backwards from each end-result goal to determine the necessary single-step goals. For example, if one of your end-result goals is to reduce the amount of saturated fats your family eats, a single-step goal might be to switch from whole or 2 percent milk to 1 percent or fat-free milk.

Write down each single-step goal. The more specific and creative you can be, the more likely you are to achieve long-term success.

Examine each single-step goal from every angle. Make sure they are all appropriate and attainable. If you come to an impasse, modify the goal. The more you can tailor your single-step goals to your lifestyle, the more likely you are to integrate them into your daily activities. They will become the building blocks of increased health and wellness.

Choose only one or two goals to implement at a time. After several weeks, add one or two more. This way you have time to adjust to and fine-tune your steps. It's natural to find yourself slipping into old patterns. This doesn't mean you have failed. A healthy lifestyle is not an all-or-nothing proposition. Reevaluate your goals. Make new ones if necessary. Many of us try to make sweeping changes and get discouraged when we do not meet our expectations. Changing lifestyle patterns is like turning an ocean liner; it can't be done quickly.

As a new mother, you have a unique opportunity to make health-enhancing choices for yourself and to establish healthy patterns for your family. As we know, children emulate their parents. The patterns established in childhood become the patterns your children take into adulthood. You can give your children the greatest gift of all: health.

Index

Exercise After Pregnancy: How to Look and Feel Your Best